The Private Rental Sector in Australia

Alan Morris · Kath Hulse · Hal Pawson

The Private Rental Sector in Australia

Living with Uncertainty

Springer

Alan Morris
University of Technology Sydney
Sydney, NSW, Australia

Kath Hulse
Swinburne University of Technology
Melbourne, VIC, Australia

Hal Pawson
University of New South Wales
Sydney, NSW, Australia

ISBN 978-981-33-6671-8 ISBN 978-981-33-6672-5 (eBook)
https://doi.org/10.1007/978-981-33-6672-5

Cover design (key designer) by eStudio Calamar, Berlin/Figueres

This Springer imprint is published by the registered company Springer Nature Singapore Pte Ltd.
The registered company address is: 152 Beach Road, #21-01/04 Gateway East, Singapore 189721, Singapore

This book is dedicated to all those individuals and families struggling to find suitable, secure and affordable rental accommodation in Australia

Preface

More than one in four Australian households, more than two million households, rent their home from a private landlord, either directly or through a real estate agent, and that number is continuing to rise. In the 20-year period, 1997–1998 to 2017–2018, the percentage of private renters increased from 20 to 27% of all households (ABS, 2019). Although it remains predominantly a transitional housing tenure for many, there is a growing cohort of long-term (ten years or more) renters, with some facing lifelong tenant status. On current estimates at least one in three private renter households are long-term renters. Most are renting privately because they are unable to access home ownership or social rental housing. This is due primarily to house price increases far outstripping income growth, more especially in Sydney and Melbourne, Australia's two largest cities, and a substantial decline of social housing as a proportion of the total housing stock.

Despite its expanding role as long-term housing, the private rental sector (PRS) is lightly regulated by Australian governments and provides tenants with little protection from eviction, other tenancy termination or rent increases. Written agreements (or leases) are usually for six or 12 months in the first instance, and usually a monthly tenancy after that. A tenant can be asked to vacate with only limited notice and in most of Australia there is no landlord obligation to give reasons for the decision. Further, rents can be increased to whatever the market can bear. The light regulation of landlord behaviour means that for low-income renters who invariably have few housing choices, everyday life can be fraught with anxiety. This unease is premised on their housing costs typically compromising their capacity to purchase necessities (rental stress), and a recognition that once their lease ends their housing situation becomes uncertain. On the other hand, some of the growing numbers of middle and higher income tenants prioritise flexibility to accommodate jobs, education or travel. For them, even Australia's relatively insecure form of private renting may be a suitable housing solution, as least for a period of time.

This book aims to provide a comprehensive understanding of the issues raised by a growing PRS where regulatory settings have remained largely unchanged since the 1980s, despite the sector's ever-increasing role in Australia's housing market. At the heart of the book is our research on tenant experiences within this setting. It is aimed at a wide readership, including the general public, media, policy-makers and other researchers. It examines the history of the sector, its financing and ownership structure and associated policy settings. A key feature is that it presents the voices of private renters, particularly those who are vulnerable by way of being outside the labour force, being of older age, having caring responsibilities and/or subsisting on low incomes. It draws on a decade of research undertaken by the authors individually and collectively on the workings of Australia's rental market.

Whilst there is an increasing array of numbers and statistics, what is often missing in accounts of private renting is the voices of the renters themselves. Chapters 4, 5, 6 and 7, draw mainly on original research (see Appendix) with long-term private renters and older renters dependent on the government Age Pension (some of the older renters interviewed were long-term renters, others had recently entered the PRS). These inform a rich and nuanced understanding of private renting from the tenant perspective. This material is complemented by findings from a representative survey of 600 private renters (including 200 long-term renters) across contrasting rental markets in inner, middle and outer suburban locations of Sydney and Melbourne.

The first chapter maps out the history of the PRS in Australia explaining its increasingly poor reputation pre-WW2, its mid-century decline and its rise over the last three decades. The policies and tax settings that helped bring about this latest resurgence are discussed. The chapter concludes by profiling the contemporary tenant population, the housing stock portfolio and its ownership. We argue that besides house prices outstripping household incomes on the demand side, a key determinant of the resurgence has been the supply side financialisation of housing in which investing in rental housing is viewed as a highly rational and desirable activity.

Chapter 2 reviews the legal frameworks that regulate the PRS in Australia, benchmarked against comparator countries. The focus is on Victoria and New South Wales. It illustrates how, by the standard of many comparator countries, current legislation provides little protection for tenants. Recent and current ongoing struggles to enhance tenants' rights are discussed.

Chapter 3 delves into the dynamics of private rental investment in Australia, examining the ownership structure and landlords' motivations, expectations and experiences. Housing financialisation is discussed as a key explanatory factor. The chapter also investigates a new actor in the sector, the institutional investor, and new investment initiatives—"build to rent", and purpose-built student housing. The rise of Airbnb and the impacts of burgeoning short-term letting are assessed.

Chapter 4 investigates the trajectory of households into the PRS. The chapter analyses the housing careers of private renters in diverse housing markets across Sydney and Melbourne. In addition, the trajectory of older people into the PRS is examined. Pathways into private renting including disruption in income, divorce and separation, fall out with children and blocked access to social housing, are discussed. Whilst most private renters would prefer to be homeowners, a growing phenomenon, especially amongst young professionals, is renting by choice. This feature is also explored in the chapter.

Finding and creating a home are key challenges for private renters. Chapter 5 examines the challenges private renters face in finding suitable and affordable accommodation and whether, once this often difficult task is accomplished, they are able to create a sense of home. Issues around landlord-tenant relations, maintenance, the condition and suitability of the accommodation and the impact of restrictions are examined.

Drawing on the in-depth interviews conducted and data from the questionnaire survey, Chapter 6 maps out the financial stress of renters in low, medium and high-rent areas in Sydney and Melbourne and the capacity of renters to lead a decent life and provide adequately for themselves and other household members. Current estimates are that about two thirds of low-income private renters (households in the bottom 40% of Australia's income distribution) experience rental stress, i.e. they need to devote more than 30% of their income to rent (Productivity Commission, 2019). The chapter also explores the impacts of rental stress on well-being focusing primarily on interviewees reliant on government benefits.

Chapter 7 investigates how secure tenants feel in their accommodation, taking into account not only legal aspects but also tenants' experiences and their perceptions of security. The focus is on low-income households whose capacity to deal with a rent increase or "notice to vacate" is often very limited.

Our final chapter, Chapter 8, besides highlighting the key findings of the study, assesses the future of the PRS in Australia. We argue that there are two potential future scenarios. The one scenario is the continuation of present trends. This will see the continued growth of the PRS, dominance of small-scale landlords and the persistence of inadequate regulation and related insecurity. The second scenario could see the private rental market permanently altered by the Covid-19 pandemic. An increase in vacancy rates may make the sector less attractive for small investors and perhaps encourage the entry of larger institutional investors. It may also force government to increase support for tenants and reduce insecurity.

Sydney, Australia — Alan Morris
Melbourne, Australia — Kath Hulse
Sydney, Australia — Hal Pawson

References

ABS (Australian Bureau of Statistics). (2019). *More households renting as home ownership falls*. Media release, 17 July. Canberra: ABS.

Productivity Commission. (2019). *Vulnerable private renters: Evidence and options*. Canberra: Commission Research Paper.

Acknowledgements

This book was totally reliant on private renters preparedness to talk about their experiences in the private rental sector. We are deeply grateful to the approximately 100 private renters who shared their stories.

We would also like to acknowledge the support of our respective research centres—the Institute for Public Policy and Governance at the University of Technology Sydney, the Centre for Urban Transitions at Swinburne University of Technology and the City Futures Research Centre at the University of New South Wales.

Funding for the study of private renters was provided by the Australian Research Council.

Finally, we would like to thank the anonymous referees and Robert Mowbray for their constructive comments and Sebastian Gutierrez-Hood for his help with the referencing. We would also like to thank Eidin O'Shea, Juliana Lobo De Queiroz and Josee Huennekes for their assistance with the conducting of the interviews and Sasindu Gamage for her help with the NVivo coding of the interviews.

Contents

About the Authors

Alan Morris is a Professor of Sociology in the Institute for Public Policy and Governance at the University of Technology Sydney. He has published extensively on housing and urban issues. His most recent books include Gentrification and Displacement: The Forced Relocation of Public Housing Tenants in Inner-Sydney (2019), The Australian Dream: Housing Experiences of Older Australians (2016) and A Practical Guide to In-depth Interviewing (2015).

Kath Hulse is Professor of Housing Studies at the Centre for Urban Transitions, Swinburne University of Technology, Melbourne. She researches and publishes on a broad range of contemporary issues which include housing market dynamics and spatial patterns of socio-economic disadvantage. Her work on the private rental sector is recognised nationally and internationally.

Hal Pawson is Professor of Housing Research and Policy, University of New South Wales, Sydney, and an Associate Director of UNSW's City Futures Research Centre. Renowned as a housing researcher both in Australia and the UK, he is also a Fellow of the Chartered Institute of Housing, and a Managing Editor of the international journal Housing Studies. He is the author of Housing Policy in Australia: A Case for System Reform (2020) with Vivienne Milligan and Judith Yates.

Abbreviations

ABS	Australian Bureau of Statistics
BtR	Build to Rent
CHC	Commonwealth Housing Commission
CRA	Commonwealth Rent Assistance
CSHA	Commonwealth-State Housing Agreement
DSP	Disability Support Pension
DSS	Department of Social Security
HILDA	Household Income and Labour Dynamics in Australia
LTR	Long-Term Renter
NSW	New South Wales
PRS	Private Rental Sector
RA	Rent Assistance
RTA	Residential Tenancies Act

Chapter 1
Back to the Future? The Decline and Rise of Private Renting in Australia

Abstract The chapter charts three main periods in the history of private renting since the end of WW1. In the first period (1919–1945), private renting was widespread in the working-class inner suburbs of Sydney and Melbourne but became deeply unpopular due to evictions and poor quality, badly maintained properties. In the second period (1946-mid-1980s), post-war reconstruction efforts supported mass home ownership and a fledgling public housing sector, and ignored the problems of private renting. Private renting declined in this new "home ownership society" until its mid-1960s nadir, attracting attention again only in the 1970s with the "rediscovery" of high levels of poverty among private renters. In the third period (mid-1980s to the present), private renting increased again due partly to tax and policy settings that stimulated investment in rental housing allied with greater demand from households unable to exit the PRS into home ownership (or public housing) as occurred in prior decades. The chapter concludes with a profile of private renting today outlining considerable diversity in the ages and household incomes of renters; long term as well as short/medium term renters; and considerable intra-city variation in rents with the lowest rents in outer suburbs.

Introduction

In the first Australian Census taken in April 1911, just under half (48%) of all households living in private dwellings were renters and just over half (52%) were recorded as home owners (Commonwealth Statistician, 1917). Fast forward to today and more than a quarter of Australian households (27%) now rent privately (ABS, 2019). While this sounds like a sector in long-term decline in what is often called a "home ownership society", the story of private renting in Australia is much more complex as we introduce in this chapter and chart throughout this book. The book examines the history of private renting in Australia, its financing and ownership structure and the ways in which government policies have shaped the sector. Importantly, it includes the voices of private renters themselves which are often missing from accounts of the sector. The book presents the diversity of private renting experiences in high, medium

A. Morris et al., *The Private Rental Sector in Australia*,
https://doi.org/10.1007/978-981-33-6672-5_1

and low rent areas of Sydney and Melbourne and highlights the perspectives of older and longer term tenants.

Existing texts on Australia's housing and urban history have said little about private renting. In this chapter, we start to fill this gap. It identifies three broad periods for private renting in modern Australia. In the first, from the end of World War 1 (WW1) to the end of World War 2 (WW2), private renting remained widespread despite concern about poor quality dwellings lacking basic amenities including adequate sanitation, which contributed to the sector's deepening unpopularity. In the second period, following WW2 and up to the early 1980s, there was a steep decline then plateauing of private renting against the backdrop of growing home ownership and public rental housing construction. In this phase, private renting fell largely under the radar of policy and media debates. In the third era, since the mid-1980s, the sector has been growing once again both numerically and proportionately—especially since the millennium. The chapter concludes with a brief profile of the contemporary private rental sector (PRS) in Australia, highlighting some aspects that differ from similar countries.

An Increasingly Unpopular Form of Housing: Private Renting 1919–1945

While private renting remained highly important in Australia after WW1, it developed a particularly bad reputation in the interwar period (1919–1939). Of particular concern was the poor quality and deteriorating condition of housing built specifically for rental in the 19th and early 20th century (Paris, 1993). A distinct stock of rental properties had been constructed in large cities such as Sydney and Melbourne, largely separated from areas of owner occupied housing. Many of these rented houses were concentrated in the then working class inner-city areas (Neutze, 1977).

These rented houses (often called cottages at the time) continued to provide housing for working class people in close proximity to the mainly small-scale industries that dominated the inner suburbs of Australia's largest cities after WW11. However, they were often poorly built and lacked even the most basic amenities including hot water and sanitation. In the interwar period, as they aged, many of these properties fell into disrepair exacerbated by a lack of maintenance as many landlords effectively disinvested from these assets (Harris, 1988). At the same time, better off residents of these inner-city areas began to move to new suburbs beyond the inner city which were developed in the interwar period (McCalman, 1993) leaving behind poorer residents with limited rent-paying capacity.

Besides these rented cottages, boarding houses were an important part of the PRS during this period. Many people lacked the means to live independently and boarded with another family or in a more formal boarding house,[1] rather than renting a whole

[1] Known as rooming houses in parts of Australia.

dwelling. Boarding houses were occupied by a broad cross section of the population and accommodated 5–10% of Melbourne and Sydney residents.

> Usually run by women, [boarding houses] provided safe and respectable shelter, daily meals, as well as laundry and other house-keeping services to a wide variety of age and social groups, and were an acceptable, even desirable form of accommodation for those without the opportunity or desire to maintain a house or flat on their own. (O'Hanlon, 2002, p. 240)

Genteel boarding houses of this type for middle and upper-class residents were different from lodging houses which provided nightly accommodation for poor and/or working class Australians of the time (O'Hanlon, 2002). As with rental properties more generally, these were often geographically concentrated. In Melbourne, for example, boarding houses were in middle class areas to the south and east areas of the city while lodging houses were to the north and west in working class areas.

The interwar period also saw the slow development of rental apartments (then universally called flats), rather than houses, as land prices rose in inner urban areas, notably in Sydney. Although generally unpopular with tenants, these were appealing to landlords as they provided a greater financial return than houses (Thompson, 1986, p. 30). The number of newly built rental flats in Sydney grew from 1164 in 1933 to 1858 in 1947 (Thompson, 1986, p. 17) at a time when there was little new housing construction due to the Great Depression of the 1930s followed by WW2.

During and after the Great Depression, high levels of unemployment and poverty meant that the working class remained largely dependent on private rental housing, much of it by then in poor shape. Landlords developed a very bad image in this period. Not only were many of their rental properties poorly maintained and relatively expensive, but their "dubious practices" included frequent evictions (Hayward, 1996). It was an era in which landlord incomes were determined by rents and capital gains were small (Paris, 1984). Landlords also had a remarkably privileged legal position vis a vis tenants. For example, they had no repairing obligations and tenants enjoyed no legal protection from unheralded demands for higher rent or summary eviction (Bradbrook, 1975).

There is limited information on the profile of private landlords during this period, but some insight is provided through the work of the Housing Investigation and Slum Abolition Board in Melbourne in 1936–37. The Board's 1937 Report controversially listed the owners of 300 houses in inner Melbourne judged "unfit for human habitation". The list "included the names of Members of Parliament, municipal councillors, estate agents and their relatives, leading business firms ... and well-known citizens" (Harris, 1988, p. 30).

A variety of individuals and organisations became concerned at perceived "slum conditions" affecting inner-city rental housing in the 1930s, a phenomenon exacerbated by the out-flow of middle-class people moving to buy detached houses in new suburbs surrounding the inner ring (McCalman, 1993), the localities we would today define as "middle suburbs". Campaigners protesting about PRS conditions were a mixed bunch. They included labour movement figures and social reformers "often with one eye on the potential threat posed by the nascent, yet growing, Australian Communist movement" (Hayward, 1996, p. 7).

Government reports of the period[2] highlighted the plight of working class slum dwelling renters in large cities. The solution was seen increasingly as providing an alternative to private landlords. This view prevailed, and State Housing Commissions were established in three states (New South Wales, Victoria and South Australia) by the end of WW2 and in the remaining three states soon afterwards. These were to provide public housing as an alternative to the PRS post WW2.

The federal government also began to take an active role in planning for post-war reconstruction (Berry, 1999). In this process, private renting was presented as a welfare problem and as contributing to urban disorder. The emotive word 'slums' was used increasingly to refer not only to housing conditions, but also to the supposed immorality and criminality of residents. Birch (2002) highlights how in Melbourne this characterisation was used to present an argument for inner-city slum housing demolition and relocation of poor families to "better" housing in other areas. The Report of the Commonwealth Committee on Social Security 1942 provides a striking illustration of official perspectives on these issues:

> Slums are at once recognized as the prime cause of disease, crime and economic wastage and a lowering of personal and civic standards. We can never hope to eradicate tuberculosis while permitting sub-standard houses without proper ventilation and sunlight, and invaded by dampness to remain, or prevent child delinquency while narrow slum streets provide the only playground for children already housed in overcrowded, insanitary and unhygienic conditions. (cited in Jones, 1972, p. 8)

In 1943, the federal government took the unprecedented step of establishing a Commonwealth Housing Commission (CHC) to make plans for post-war reconstruction. The Commission saw the housing problem as part of a broader urban policy challenge rather than as a welfare issue. In its Final Report, it scathingly indicted the failure of the private market to provide adequate and affordable rental housing for workers (Commonwealth Housing Commission, 1944, p. 17, clause 99). It also argued that housing should not be used to generate excessive profits for landlords:

> The Commission considers that the housing of the people of the Commonwealth adequately, soundly, hygienically, and effectively, each according to his social and economic life is a national need, and, accordingly, should cease to be a field of investment yielding high profits. (Commonwealth Housing Commission, 1944, p. 18, clause 98)

To address an acute housing shortage, including both pent-up demand and substandard rental property in need of replacement post WW2, the CHC recommended that the federal government negotiate with the states to establish a significant public rental house-building program[3] and provide assistance to people to buy their own homes. It did not include any strategies to improve private rental housing; the PRS

---

[2]Reports included the Report of the Victorian Government's Housing Investigation and Slum Abolition Board (1936), the Housing Slums Investigation Committee of the NSW Parliament (1936) and the Building Act Inquiry Committee of the SA Government (1937).

[3]The Commission recommended that rents for Commonwealth-financed public housing of an agreed adequate standard should be the economic rent or one sixth of the family income, whatever is the less (1944, p. 13, clause 48).

was seen as the problem to be addressed and not as part of the solution to the extreme housing shortage in the early post-war period. As a result, the PRS remained virtually unregulated until the late 1970s as we shall see in the next section.

Private Renting from WW2 to the Early 1980s: A Declining and Forgotten Sector

The Decline of Private Renting and the Rise of Home Ownership and Public Housing

The quarter century after WW2 (1945–1970) saw a steady decline in private renting as more households became home owners or rented from the newly established State Housing Commissions, although public housing never exceeded 6% of all housing across Australia (see Fig. 1.1). The "long boom" enjoyed during this period featured high economic growth and low unemployment which, along with direct government support (Pawson et al., 2020), enabled a rapid increase in home ownership in the decades to 1970 (Berry, 1999). In consequence, the home ownership rate increased from 53% in 1947 to a high of 71% in 1966 (Kryger, 2009).

The 1945 Commonwealth-State Housing Agreement (CSHA) also provided federal funding for the first time for a public housing program with housing built and managed by the states; between 1945 and 1971 one in ten homes were constructed with CSHA funds (Neutze, 1977, p. 167). Many were built for sale, or after being initially rented out were subsequently sold to residents at concessional rates in the 1950s, 1960s and 1970s.[4] Promotion of home ownership was a signature policy during the 18 years of federal governments (1949–1966) led by Robert Menzies. In a famous speech broadcast on radio in 1942 on "The Forgotten People", Menzies then in Opposition, had outlined the importance of saving to purchase a "home" equating home with family, aspiration and achievement:

> My home is where my wife and children are. The instinct to be with them is the great instinct of civilised man; the instinct to give them a chance in life - to make them not leaners but lifters - is a noble instinct. (Menzies, 1942)

As a result of these widespread sales programs, public rental housing in Australia never exceeded an estimated 6%[5] of all private occupied dwellings at any one time unlike many of European countries where public rental housing became a key part of post WW2 reconstruction. Failure to reform the PRS in this period meant that home

[4]Half of all public rental dwellings constructed with CSHA funds had been sold by 1973. The percentage of public housing stock sold varied across the states with four states having sold more than half of these dwellings: Tasmania (67.1%); Queensland (59.3%); Western Australia (59.1%); South Australia (52.6%). Victoria had sold 45.8% of its dwellings and NSW the lowest percentage at 38.3% (Neutze, 1977, p. 168).

[5]Hayward (1996) says that the maximum was 8% but this cannot be validated.

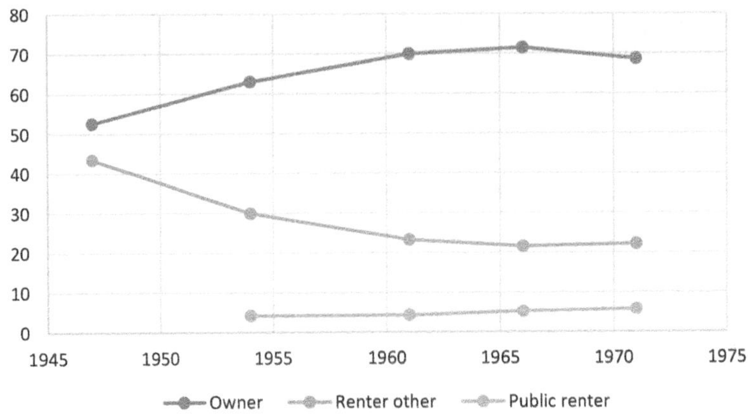

Fig. 1.1 % of occupied private dwellings by tenure type, Australia, 1945–1971 (*Source* Adapted from Neutze 1977: Table 6.9, p. 153 from Census collections in 1947, 1954, 1961, 1966, and 1971. *Note* Private renters were classified as "renter other" to distinguish them from public housing renters. "Other tenure type" is not illustrated. Tenure not stated not included in calculation of percentages)

ownership and public rental housing offered better conditions and considerably more security and control for households than private renting (Fig. 1.1).

Other factors contributing to private rental decline in the decades after WW2 included the continuation of wartime rent controls which limited returns to private landlords, and the higher interest rates charged for mortgages taken out by landlords/non-occupiers (Neutze, 1978).

The federal government had introduced wartime rent controls (the National Security [Fair Rents] Regulations in 1939) which were rolled out across most states. These controls persisted after WW2, with tenancies protected and rents often pegged at least initially at 1939 levels, making rental properties an uneconomic proposition for landlords, many of whom sold their property to the sitting tenant (Kendig, 1979). Rent controls were phased out progressively in the 1950s and 1960s (Mowbray, 1996).

Landlord incentives and returns were also depressed by penalty interest rates on mortgages for rental housing acquisition. In stark contrast, home owners benefited from regulated interest rates (Berry, 1999), which continued until the federal government-led deregulation of housing finance in the mid-1980s (Hulse et al., 2012), discussed later in this chapter.

Boarding houses, too, continued their long decline in the decades after WW2 (CURA, 1979; O'Hanlon, 2002; Dalton et al., 2015). The introduction of strata titling[6] in the 1960s which started in New South Wales (NSW) in 1961, enabled a boom in rental apartment construction in large cities. In conjunction with rising

[6]Strata titles were an Australian invention which enabled individual ownership of apartments within a multi-unit building with a owners' body corporate for management and maintenance of the common areas of the building such as roofs, external walls, stairwells and gardens. Before this, buildings were mainly owned and managed through a company structure.

incomes, this expanded opportunities for single people to rent self-contained accommodation rather than needing to rely on shared facilities in a boarding house (Dalton et al., 2015). Boarding houses became progressively associated with low-income and marginalised residents, a trend which was intensified by the de-institutionalisation of large psychiatric and disability institutions from the 1970s (Greenhalgh et al., 2004).

Gentrification and Slum Clearance

A further explanation for PRS decline from the late 1950s was inner-city gentrification. As the post-war era wore on, many such suburbs began to regain or acquire status as desirable localities. Middle class households bought rental properties in inner-city working class areas and renovated them for their own occupation, thus displacing tenants. Indeed, both here and in other countries such as the UK, conversion from private rental to resident home-ownership was viewed as a key indicator of post-war gentrification. An additional Australian factor was the arrival of southern European migrants accustomed to buying rather than renting, and their attraction to inner urban areas replete with upgradeable housing (Logan, 1985).

State Government Housing Commissions also contributed by declaring a substantial proportion of inner-city private rental housing as sub-standard and earmarking selected areas for demolition and redevelopment as part of "slum clearance" programs (from the 1960s to the mid-1970s). Such tracts were intended to be replaced with public housing, including the high rise tower blocks which still dominate the skyline of Melbourne today. While the level of amenity offered to renters in these estates was typically far better than the houses demolished, there was concern that clearance and relocation broke up some established working class communities (see for example, Birch, 2002). As the 1970s progressed, community resistance increased and this type of redevelopment by State Housing Commissions was stopped by union and community campaigns, notably in Sydney and Melbourne (Tibbits, 1988; Burgmann & Burgmann, 2017).

More intensive activity in inner cities, including the apartment boom of the late 1960s and early 1970s, led to higher land prices in these areas which, in turn, led to owners considering other, higher value uses. This affected not only cottage-style properties but also boarding houses with owners selling or repurposing them as backpacker hostels, single family residences, luxury apartments and tourist accommodation which yielded a higher return (Greenhalgh et al., 2004).

Private Renting and Poverty

The perception that the challenge of slum rental housing had been overcome turned policy and media attention from poor housing to poor people, prompted by the "rediscovery" of poverty in urban Australia in the early 1970s. A pioneering survey of Melbourne in the late 1960s had highlighted the continued existence of poverty in an age of growing affluence (Henderson et al., 1970). While the research focused on measuring the adequacy of incomes to meet basic living standards, it also acknowledged broader dimensions of poverty beyond income. Study leader, Professor Henderson, went on to chair the subsequent Federal Government Commission of Inquiry into Poverty (1972–1975) which raised the alarm about high rates of poverty among older people and large families and among private renters (Commission of Inquiry into Poverty, 1975a). It identified private renters as the group whose situation deteriorated most when comparing before and after housing costs. Private renters, moreover, accounted for 41% of all those living in (after-housing) poverty. The First Main Report of the Commission of Inquiry into Poverty (1975a) also recognised that private renters experienced problems beyond lack of affordability—including insecurity which we consider further in Chapter 7. The report cites a submission from the Glebe Residents Group in inner-Sydney on the effects of gentrification on insecurity:

> This problem of insecurity of tenure of housing in Glebe is on the increase, as the area is increasing greatly in value, and is becoming increasingly popular as a residence for the affluent. Developers and individuals are taking advantage of this to make large profits. The problem is especially serious for the low income earner and the aged and invalid [sic]. (cited in Commission of Inquiry into Poverty, 1975a, p. 161)

The Commission did original research into the situation of low-income private renters in the inner Melbourne suburbs of Fitzroy and Collingwood. Identified problems included a lack of accommodation suitable for larger families, leading to overcrowding, a lack of "social space", limited facilities such as laundry facilities, poor property condition including dampness and draughts, problems with plumbing, inadequate heating, and a lack of storage for clothes (Commission of Inquiry into Poverty, 1975c, pp. 89–92).

The Commission's First Main Report recommended income supplements (and tax credits) for low-income households, who would then rent or buy, at market prices, from a diverse range of social housing providers or in the private market, with some federal funding of supply subsidies for non-profit housing (Commission of Inquiry into Poverty, 1975a, 176–77). Other measures to stimulate or subsidise the private rental market were considered unnecessary. These recommendations had a longer-term effect in reframing the "housing problem" as primarily one of "affordability", as we discuss later in this chapter.

One important effect of the Commission's work was to apply a blowtorch to regulation of the landlord-tenant relations. In an associated report, current legislation was described as "a scandal" demanding wide-ranging reform for tenant protection (Bradbrook, 1975, p. 2). The report argued that the legislation remained based on common law which had developed in the agricultural era of eighteenth century England and was later applied inappropriately to rental buildings in urban settings in the UK and Australia. This led to many injustices for tenants. Such concerns included the lack of a landlord repairing obligation, the absence of a requirement to provide the premises in a clean condition; the lack of control over excessive rents;

the failure to apply traditional contractual principles such as mitigation of damages, frustration and repudiation; and inadequate safeguards in respect of assignment of leases to other tenant and sub-leases.

The Second Main Report of the Commission on *Poverty and the Law in Australia*, (Commission of Inquiry into Poverty (1975b) led by Professor Sackville responded in part to the research report, notably in its key recommendation that each Australian state and territory should introduce new codified legislation applicable to residential tenancies.[7] This work triggered an extended period of specialised residential tenancies legislation beginning in South Australia (1978) and followed by Victoria (1980), NSW (1987), Western Australia (1987) and Queensland (1994). However, in implementation, the extent of contestation about residential tenancies legislation enactment and the role of interest groups became apparent.

> Because of the novelty and far-reaching nature of many of the recommendations, many groups and individuals, particularly real estate agents, were deeply suspicious of the proposed reforms. For this reason the full range of reforms recommended by the Poverty Inquiry were never introduced into law in any jurisdiction. (Bradbrook, 1998, p. 405)

Bradbrook (1998), in reviewing this period, considered that some of the most important omissions from the legislation were around controlling excessive rents and rent increases and the continuation of termination without "just cause". We examine the cumulative effect of successive periods of legislative reform when considering contemporary regulation of the PRS in Chapter 2.

While there was substantial research into private renters and poverty, discussed above, relatively little is known about private landlords in the 1960s, 1970s and 1980s. In what was essentially the first review of private renting since WW2, Paris (1984) suggested that the PRS in Australia comprised temporary landlords, individual investors, corporate investors, owner-managers and informal landlords, indicating a variety of landlords and motivations. Only two of these were seen as "investors": affluent individuals who took a hands-off approach to their rental properties (such as "Sydney pilots") and corporate investors who owned rental apartments. The rest were somewhat "accidental landlords" who were amateurs in the business of renting out properties.

By the mid-1980s, one in five Australian households rented their housing on the private market, a percentage that had been stable since the mid-1960s. Australia experienced high rates of migration-fuelled population growth during this period, so the number of PRS properties did increase. In this respect, Australia differs from countries such as the UK where the number of PRS properties continued to contract throughout the post-war period until the early 1990s. A noteworthy shift was that private renters were no longer predominantly working-class families, most of whom had become home owners or moved into public rental housing. The bulk of private renters were now young people who rented for a transitional period after they left the family home, those unable to buy such as single parents and recent migrants to Australia or from within Australia (Paris, 1984). It looked as though private renting

[7] Chapter 3 of the Second Main Report was on residential tenancies law (Commission of Inquiry into Poverty, 1975b).

would remain at about a fifth of all private properties to meet these needs. These assumptions proved unfounded, as we shall discuss next, with the growth and transformation of private renting from the mid 1980s, but with a legacy of some important unresolved problems continuing to affect some of those living in private rental, particularly those on lower incomes.

The Growth of the PRS from the Mid-1980s

The mid-1980s saw key changes to Australian policy settings that contributed, sometimes incidentally, to the subsequently rapid growth in private renting. This was accompanied by a shift in the government rhetoric around private renting, with a more explicit pro-market articulation of the proposed benefits of the sector. These included the argument that the PRS provides consumer choice, offering accommodation of different types at different rent levels and in a range of locations, all seen as advantageous relative to a public rental housing model. In1995, in his Community and Nation Statement, then Labor Prime Minister Keating signalled this view of the PRS and the role of what was then called Commonwealth Rent Assistance (CRA) when he stated the way to "reduce the public housing waiting lists [is] by improving the scope for people to choose private rental accommodation" (cited in Wilkinson, 2005, p. 25). This pro-market rhetoric was further ramped up by the right of centre Coalition[8] federal government (1996–2007) which oversaw decreased funding to public housing which in consequence became strictly rationed to those with the most urgent and complex needs. In this way, private renting was more assertively proposed as providing essential housing for lower income as well as other groups, facilitated by a redirection of federal government financial support away from public housing provision to rent assistance.[9]

The reference to (Commonwealth) Rent Assistance as a means of improving affordability for private renters was part of a decades-long process in which a little-known income supplement for single pensioners who rented their housing developed incrementally into the major form of housing assistance in Australia, such that by the mid-1990s, government expenditure on RA exceeded that on social housing supply. Box 1 illustrates some of the major changes.

---

[8]A Coalition government at the federal level in Australia is made up of the right of centre Liberal Party and the National Party. The latter is a conservative party that is based in regional Australia.

[9]'Under the long-term reforms, it is proposed that the Commonwealth, instead of providing capital funding under the Commonwealth State Housing Agreement, would pay rent assistance to clients in the private and public rental structure' (DSS, 1996)

Box 1: Evolution of Rent Assistance (RA) for private renters

Postwar to early 1980s

RA originated in 1958 (then called supplementary assistance) as a small flat rate supplement for single pensioners who could not share their housing costs with another person. It was introduced as a less costly alternative to a general pension increase (Kewley, 1973). The payment was extended to couple pensioners and renamed as supplementary rent assistance in 1970 (Prosser & Leeper, 1994). This type of payment was in line with the Poverty Inquiry's recommendation of income supplements as a means of addressing poverty amongst private renters (Commission of Inquiry into Poverty, 1975a, pp. 176–177).

By the early 1980s, RA had been extended beyond the original groups of pensioners to lone parents on supporting parent's benefit and some long-term sickness beneficiaries (DSS, 1985, pp. 120–121). The flat rate payment was changed to a model with a minimum rent threshold payment of 50 cents in the dollar of the amount between this threshold and rent paid, with the amount capped by a new maximum level, a formula that has been retained with modifications ever since.

Mid-1980s to present

The incoming Labor government in 1983 was initially pro public housing but conceded that RA was a quicker means of reaching more households more quickly. In this it was buttressed by its Social Security Review (1986–7) arguing strongly that RA was more likely to ameliorate housing and poverty problems than supply side measures (Vipond, 1987, p. 2). Eligibility for the payment (renamed as Rent Assistance in 1985) was extended to most pensioners and beneficiaries and those on family payments. In just four years (1984–1988) the number of RA recipients increased from 479,998 to 713,355 recipients) (DSS, various years). Subsequent changes were made by the Labor governments (in power until 1996) to target RA more effectively to two groups: those paying higher rents and households with dependent children, changes which added to the complexity of the RA payment. Twice yearly indexation of RA payments by the Consumer Price Index was introduced in 1991 (Ey, 2012). The number of RA recipients continued to increase particularly in the recession of the early 1990s when more people were on income support payments.

The Coalition government in 1996 took a more explicitly pro-market view, arguing that the private rental market was responsive to household demand and the federal government's role was primarily to provide some assistance with rental affordability through RA. More changes were made to eligibility and further tweaking of the payment, notably a reduction in payment for single people sharing their housing (1997). This approach persisted through changes of federal government to the present. By June 2019, almost 1.3 million people and families were in receipt of RA at an annual cost of $4.4 billion (DSS, 2019, p. 94).

RA has generated several criticisms. The effective value of RA has been substantially eroded over time due to indexation using the Consumer Price Index rather than housing rent inflation (generally higher) (Productivity Commission, 2017). RA is still attached to income support payments and family tax benefits rendering low-income singles and couples on low wages ineligible for this assistance (Hulse, 2002). A further concern is that, since no conditions are imposed on landlords of recipient tenants, RA does not address longstanding concerns over quality and tenure insecurity in the private rental market outlined in this chapter.

Four key factors have contributed to post-1980s PRS growth—housing finance deregulation, the favourable tax regime for investors, the growing affordability barriers to home ownership and the relative decline of social housing. The first two of these factors relate to the *supply side* influences—conditions that encouraged private rental property investment. The third and fourth factors relate to changes that have inflated *demand* for private rental housing. These are discussed in turn.

Housing Finance Deregulation and the Favourable Tax Regime for Private Investors

During the 1980s, the federal government opened up the Australian economy to global flows of capital and labour. Financial systems, including housing finance, were deregulated as part of this process (Banks, 2004). These changes had the effect of removing the 'protected circuit' of finance for home ownership (Berry, 1999) including removal of regulated interest rates for purchasers and interest rate penalties for mortgages taken out by non-owner occupiers, who became known as rental investors, easing access to mortgages for rental property acquisition (Hulse et al., 2012, pp. 17–19). Put simply, it became easier for landlords to borrow money to acquire private rental properties.

They could also borrow more money because it was cheaper. Changing interest rates reflect global factors as well as Australian domestic influences. The average standard rate for a variable mortgage peaked at 17% in 1989/1990 before dropping rapidly to 6% at the end of the 20th century. In the new century, rates increased to 9.45% just before the GFC in 2008 and have generally declined since to lows of 5% in 2019, rates not seen since the late 1950s (Whitten, 2020). This "cheap money" enabled landlords to borrow more to purchase their rental properties.

The tax regime also encouraged the expansion of private landlordism. Negative gearing—the capacity to deduct any losses from a rental property from entire taxable income—makes rental property investment extremely attractive for salaried individuals, particularly those in higher paid employment. This long-standing tax provision from the 1920s was little known until the government removed it in 1985, but reinstated it in 1987 following extensive lobbying by the real estate industry (Hulse & Burke, 2015). This had the effect of highlighting its existence and attractiveness to many more landlords and potential landlords. In addition, the capital gains tax regime is also very favourable for investors including private landlords. Under a provision enacted in 1999, a rental property held for more than 12 months incurs tax on only 50% of the landlord's nominal capital gain (Daly & Wood, 2016). In the big housing price inflation which followed the recession of the early 1990s, these tax benefits were of increasing importance, as discussed in more detail in Chapter 3.

Deregulation of housing finance, increased knowledge of tax incentives and access to cheap money in combination contributed to an increase in private rental supply from the 1980s. This is part of what has been termed the "financialisation of housing" (Aalbers, 2016; Fainstein, 2016), connecting ordinary households to money flows in the global economy. There were, however, also social and cultural reasons for the rise of private landlords including viewing housing as an asset and an investment rather than somewhere to live. Much on the commentary on this is negative:

> Housing is under attack today ... Most immediately, there is a conflict between housing as lived, social space and housing as an instrument for profitmaking-a conflict between housing as *home* and as *real estate.* (Madden & Marcuse, 2016, p. 4, italics in original).

Other commentators have pointed to the rise of asset-based welfare; households were encouraged to fund their own welfare needs through asset accumulation and draw-down rather than rely on government welfare as a reason for becoming landlords (Ronald & Kadi, 2018).

Affordability Barriers to Home Ownership and the Relative Decline of Social Housing

Demand for private rental also rose as other alternatives became less accessible, namely home ownership and social rented housing. On the first of these, there has been much commentary about the affordability problems facing potential home owners since the mid-1980s and particularly since the late 1990s as housing prices began to increase rapidly. Residential property price increases in Australia, more especially in Sydney and Melbourne, began to far outstrip increases in income. The Parliamentary library calculated that between June 1981 and June 2015, the "ratio of average disposable income (Australia-wide) to median house prices … increased from approximately 3.3 to just over 7 …" (Thomas & Hall, 2016). Later, between 2012 and 2017, house prices in Sydney increased by 75% and in Melbourne by 58% (Wright, 2019). The surge in residential property prices has resulted in a substantial proportion of individuals/households being unable to access home ownership. For most, the PRS is their only alternative.

The single most important driver of post-1990s house price inflation has probably been the long term decline in mortgage interest rates seen over that period. In the 25 years to 2020, the standard variable rate for an owner occupier loan fell by half to 5% (RBA, 2020), substantially increasing the size of a mortgage supportable on any given income and, therefore, the amount prospective purchasers have felt they are able to offer to property vendors.

Other factors include rising real wages, the greater purchasing power associated with the rise of two income households and competition from landlords (both local and foreign) for the same properties. Tax privileged and cashed up landlords can often outbid low-moderate income and younger households who then have little option but to rent (Morris, 2018). As rents have also risen this has made it more difficult for private renters, not only in terms of meeting current housing costs, but also in saving for a house purchase deposit. This would appear to be a rather vicious circle that is difficult to break.

Of course, there are also other reasons why the past 20–30 years have seen additional demand for private renting. People up to their mid-30s rented privately for various reasons including the growth of contract and casual employment that may have impaired their creditworthiness and or capacity to save for a deposit (Burke et al., 2020). Other reasons include deferral of home purchase due to a preference for study and travel and later partnering and parenting (Simon & Stone, 2017).

At the bottom end of the market, growing numbers of low-income households were increasingly unable to access a stagnant public housing sector which was unable to cater for anyone beyond "highest need" applicants (Pawson et al., 2020). These trends have contributed to an increase in lower-income private renters (Wulff et al., 2011) as well as a newly identified phenomenon of long-term renters, those renting for more than 10 years (first identified by Wulff & Maher, 1998).

Initially, alongside its moves to deregulate housing finance, the Hawke Labor government (elected in 1983) pledged to increase public rental housing. In the decade, 1985 to 1995, about 115,000 such properties were built, boosting national stock to 388,600 in 1995 (McIntosh, 1997). At this rate of increase, public housing provision was more-or-less keeping pace with overall population growth. Waiting lists nevertheless continued to expand, growing from 145,000 in 1985 to 235,000 by 1995 (McIntosh, 1997). Subsequently, the election of the Howard Coalition government in 1996, saw the effective end of a routine public house-building program in Australia and accessing social housing became exceptionally difficult, reserved for applicants with complex needs. According to the Productivity Commission (2018), the gross number of social housing lettings nationally dropped from 52,000 in 1997 to 35,000 in 2017. While this represents an absolute decline of a third, pro rata to population the effective reduction in social housing supply was 50%.

Summarising these changes to supply and demand for private renting, it is clear that private renting has bounced back from its post-war low in 1966 with slow growth to the mid-1990s followed by more rapid expansion thereafter. In 2018, around 27% of Australian households were private renters, up from 18% in 1994. Largely at the expense of owner occupation, PRS growth was particularly strong in the first two decades of the 21st century, as shown in Fig. 1.2.

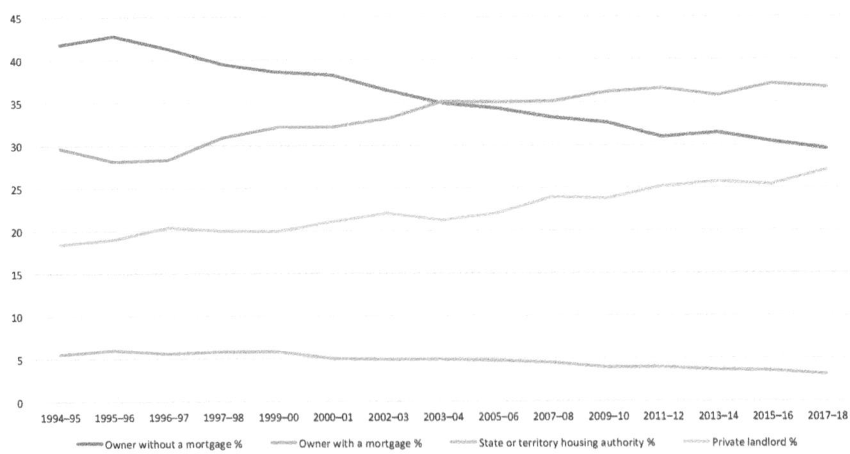

Fig. 1.2 Changes in housing tenure, Australia, 1994–95 to 2017–18 (*Source* Calculated from ABS 2019, Table 1. *Note* Data from ABS Housing Occupancy and Costs series gives a slightly higher percentage of private rental than the ABS Census, however, the data are comparable across the years included)

The growth in the PRS reflects broader changes in Australia's society and economy. However, this story is not unique to Australia. Comparative research has identified PRS growth in countries which are somewhat similar to Australia, particularly New Zealand, the UK, the US and Ireland (Whitehead et al., 2012; Crook & Kemp, 2014; Martin et al., 2018). It is important to note that growth does not simply mean more of the same as we discuss next.

A Profile of the Contemporary Private Rental Sector

We conclude this brief history of the PRS by providing a contemporary profile of the sector. This provides context for the discussion of regulation and policy that follows in Chapters 2 and 3.

Who Lives in the Sector?

In 2016, just over four in ten private renters (42%) were younger households (15–34 years), a considerably lower percentage than the 55% recorded in 1996. Specifically, the percentage of young renters aged 15–24 years has halved over this period and the proportion of renters aged 25–34 has declined modestly, but still represents just under a third (32%) of all private renters (see Table 1.1). This accords with research which highlights that greater numbers of younger people are remaining in their family home until their late 20 s or rent privately for a period and then return

Table 1.1 Private renters and all households by age 1996, 2006, 2016

	1996		2006		2016	
	Private renters	All households	Private renters	All households	Private renters	All households
Age (years)	%	%	%	%	%	%
15–24	20	6	14	5	10	4
25–34	35	19	31	16	32	16
35–44	23	23	24	21	24	19
45–54	18	32	16	21	17	20
55–64			9	16	10	17
65+	5	20	6	21	7	25
Total	100	100	100	100	100	100

Source Hulse et al. (2019: Tables 7 and A10), Yates et al. (2004: Table 4.1). *Notes* Age refers to age of household head; may not add up to 100% due to rounding

home (Wilkins & Vera-Toscano, 2019).[10] The percentage of renters aged 45–64 years, in contrast, increased from 18 to 27% in the 20 years to 2016.

There has also been a modest increase in the proportion of older (65+ years) private renters—Table 1.1. While their representation remains relatively small, the 163,000 private tenant households in this cohort considerably exceeded the 115,000 older households who rented public housing in 2016. This position has reversed since 1996 when older private renters numbered 62,000 households—far fewer than the number living in public rental housing who have controlled rents and greater security. This trend is likely to accelerate over coming decades, as older persons' home ownership rates decline (Coates & Chen, 2019). These changes suggest that PRS growth is fuelled mainly by mid-life and older households unable to exit the PRS into home ownership (or social housing) as occurred in previous decades, rather than by the entry of new, younger households into private renting. In consequence, the percentage of long-term renters (10 years or more) increased from 27% in 1996 to 33% in 2011 (Stone et al., 2013).

There has been some change in the PRS household type profile over the period 1996–2016. The percentage of young people living alone and in group households (typically comprising young people) declined from 35% of private renters in 1996 to 25% in 2016. Conversely, the proportion of couple households at all ages increased from 41% in 1996 to 47% in 2016. The percentage of households with children had increased prior to 1996 and remains high—about 40% of all private renters (Hulse et al. 2019, Table 7 and Table A10).

The PRS houses many lower income households including those unable to access social rental housing. It is, however, a very diverse sector and there has been an increase of middle and higher income private renters over the two decades to 2016, as illustrated in Fig. 1.3.

The *number* of households earning under $42,000 p.a. in $2016 has remained stable at about 500,000 over the past 20 years[11] (Hulse et al., 2019, p. 29). However, when we use quintiles, which is a relative measure of the distribution of all Australian household incomes, the numbers of households in the lowest and second lowest quintiles in the PRS have increased along with sector growth.[12] It is for this reason that a recent report by the federal government's Productivity Commission found

[10] The research used longitudinal data from the Household Income and Labour Dynamics of Australia (HILDA) survey. It found that in 2017, 56% of men aged 18–29 lived with one or both parents, up from 47% in 2001 and the proportion of women aged 18–29 living with their parents rose from 36 to 54% over the same period (Wilkins and Vera-Toscano, 2019).

[11] The poverty line for the September quarter in 2016 inclusive of housing costs for a family constituting two adults and two dependent children was $967.23 a week or $50,296 a year (Melbourne Institute, 2016).

[12] Between 2006 and 2016, the number of PRS households grew by 38 per cent (or 553,000 households), more than twice the rate of growth of all Australian households (16%). In the same decade, the number of lowest quintile private rental households grew by 30% (80,000 households) and the second lowest quintile households by 32% (116,000 households), each roughly twice the rate of all households (calculated from Hulse et al., 2019, p. 99, Table A3).

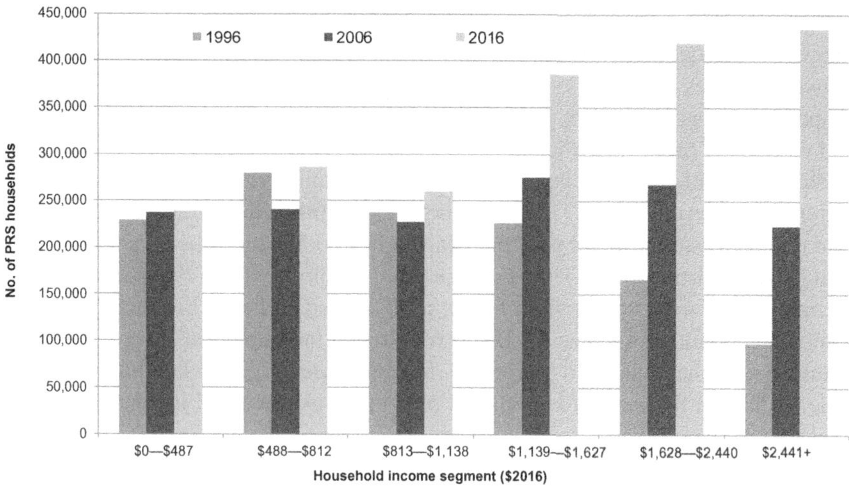

Fig. 1.3 Household weekly income of private renter households, Australia, 1996–2016 (*Source* Adapted from Hulse et al. [2019, figure 7], with additional data for 1996 from prior project in the series. *Note* Household income figures are all in 2016 dollars and comparable in real terms. Figures refer to real change in constant dollars and the household income segments are not quantiles [such as quintiles or quartiles])

that the PRS is increasingly important as the main means of accommodating low-income households including those that are vulnerable (Productivity Commission, 2019, p. 42). These include single parent households on low incomes, a group often unable to access social housing unless gaining priority due to urgent and complex needs.

It is also important to note that the incidence of private renting varies across Australia. More than a third of households are private renters in Darwin, Brisbane and Sydney. Representation is lower in Melbourne, Adelaide, Hobart and Perth (Rowley & James, 2018). There are higher rates of private renting in Queensland and Western Australia with their mining towns and in the two territories (ACT and Northern Territory) than in Victoria, Tasmania and South Australia.

Who Owns and Manages Australia's Privately Rented Properties?

2.03 million individual taxpayers—nearly 16% of all Australian taxpayers—owned at least a share in a rental property in 2015–16 up from 10% in 2003–04 (CoreLogic, 2016; Hulse et al., 2019). At a household level, 13.8% of households own properties for which they receive regular rent payment, up from 10% in 2003–04, the first year in which such data were collected (Hulse et al., 2019, p. 10). Interestingly, some households occupying rental dwellings themselves are also landlords, about one in eight such tenants across Australia (Hulse & McPherson, 2014), a group sometimes known by the real estate industry-coined term, *rentvestors*. Most landlords have one or two properties but there is some evidence of an increase in landlords with multiple properties (Hulse et al., 2019, p. 11). Chapter 3 provides further detail about landlords and patterns of property ownership.

What is significant here, beyond the increase in numbers of landlords and the size of rental property holdings, is the discursive reframing of landlords as "Mum and Dad rental investors", thereby normalising and valorising this type of activity (Hulse et al., 2019; Martin, 2018). This is a huge change from the much-derided landlord of the interwar years, a semi-pariah figure, as discussed earlier in this chapter. Unlike some other countries such as the US, private rental investment in Australia remains dominated by the household sector and, to date, large corporate landlords have had little traction in the mainstream market although—as discussed in Chapter 3—this may change in coming years.

A further change is the extent to which landlords use rental property managers to handle their properties and tenants. Seven in ten privately rented properties in Australia are managed by real estate agents (Martin et al., 2018) such that most landlords are hands-off in terms of management of their properties and addressing renter concerns. Agent responsiveness has become a key issue in thinking about the future of private renting. In relying on intermediaries in this way, the Australian PRS differs from some other countries, particularly in Europe, where direct management by the landlord remains more common (Martin et al., 2018). Recent national surveys of private renters have highlighted some management issues associated with the PRS including discrimination against those with children, being in receipt of government benefits, having certain ethnic backgrounds (Rowley & James, 2018; Choice et al., 2017) and owning pets (Power, 2017).

What Are the Characteristics of Private Rental Properties?

Recent comparative research has highlighted that the Australian PRS is less differentiated from the rest of the housing market than in many comparator countries. This is true in relation to property types, as well as the demographic characteristics of tenants (Martin et al., 2018). That is, PRS properties are generally not identifiable by their physical form. In many comparable countries, the bulk of private rental accommodation is apartments. In Australia, however, half of private renters (52%) live in a detached (separate) house and only 27% live in an apartment (Hulse et al., 2019). Nevertheless, somewhat fewer private renters live in separate houses and more in flats/apartments than for Australian households generally. This is particularly the case in Sydney and to a lesser extent in Melbourne and Brisbane. There is also evidence of a bifurcated market within large cities: with an inner-city apartment rental market and the middle-outer suburban house rental market.

Private rents have been increasingly concentrated at levels affordable to middle and higher income households rather than lower income earners (Hulse et al., 2019;

Productivity Commission, 2019). As a corollary, there have been growing shortages for those on very low and low incomes (Hulse et al., 2019) as discussed further in Chapter 6. More affordable (less expensive) rentals are increasingly located in the outer suburbs of major cities, peri-urban areas and regional areas where land values are lower. These areas are often poorly served by public transport and remote from centres of employment and services. This is a complete turnaround from the situation up to the mid-1970s, when private rented properties and low-income populations were concentrated in inner-city areas as discussed earlier.

Conclusion

The history of private renting in Australia provides essential insights into the evolution of the nation's housing system, and the resulting implications for the life chances of today's Australians. In this chapter, we have shown how a sector that was a mainstream housing option became increasingly unpopular after WW1 and during the Great Depression due to poor quality properties, deteriorating conditions and unscrupulous landlords. In the early post-WW2 era reforming the PRS to address these concerns was not part of the imaginary of reconstruction to make a better world. Rather private renting had become associated with a dark past and there was now a desire to do something different. The something different was extensive policy support for working class families to own their own homes and to build public housing for either rent or sale. In this context, the PRS contracted in the mid-twentieth century as home ownership grew to accommodate just over 70% of households and a modest but important public housing sector was established.

These settings were shaken in the 1970s by the rediscovery of poverty, notwithstanding Australia's long post-war economic boom. Importantly, Australian households who rented privately at the nadir of the sector had very high rates of poverty after paying for their housing, as well as experiencing a range of other problems including poor property condition and quality and a lack of security. As a result, specific residential tenancies legislation was introduced by the Australian states to replace the "scandal" of landlord-tenant regulation which derived from feudal relations in eighteenth century England. There have been several waves of state legislative change since 1975 but, as further discussed in Chapter 2, a good deal of continuity. Thus most states currently continue to permit eviction without "just cause". Survey data suggest that limited amenities and poor condition at the low rent end of the market remain a problem as well as some aspects of management of properties.

The PRS increased its share of the Australian housing system slowly from the mid-1980s and has experienced something of a resurgence since the start of the 21st century. This chapter has documented some of the reasons why this has occurred, including the rise of small-scale private landlords who have been able to borrow money to fund their purchases in a deregulated housing finance system supported by tax incentives. It has also outlined why demand for private rental has increased as home purchase has become unaffordable for some and the option of social rental housing has been increasingly severely rationed. The sector now houses more than a quarter of all Australian households. Private renters are increasingly diverse including renters at midlife and in older age as well as younger households. Middle and higher income households, as well as their poorer counterparts, are also well-represented. In the next chapter we examine how regulation has responded to some of these changes.

References

Aalbers, M. B. (2016). *The financialization of housing: A political economy approach.* New York: Routledge.

ABS (Australian Bureau of Statistics). (2019). Housing occupancy and costs 2017–18, Cat, No. 4130.0. Canberra: ABS Canberra. https://www.abs.gov.au/ausstats/abs@.nsf/exnote/4130.0.

Banks, G. (2004). Structural reform Australian-style: Lessons for others? *Economic Survey of Australia, 2004.* Paris: OECD (Organisation of Economic Co-Operation and Development). https://www.oecd.org/australia/39218531.pdf.

Berry, M. (1999). Unravelling the "Australian Housing Solution": The Post-War years. *Housing, Theory and Society, 16*(3), 106–123.

Birch, A. (2002). *Framing Fitzroy: Contesting and (de)constructing place and identity in a Melbourne suburb.* PhD thesis, Department of History, The University of Melbourne (unpublished). http://minerva-access.unimelb.edu.au/handle/11343/36250.

Bradbrook, A. J. (1975). *Poverty and the residential landlord-tenant relationship.* Canberra: Australian Government Publishing Service.

Bradbrook, A. J. (1998). Residential tenancies law—The second stage of reforms. *Sydney Law Review, 20*(3), 402–434.

Burgmann, M., & Burgmann, V. (2017). *Green bans, red unfion.* Sydney: UNSW Press.

Burke, T., Nygaard, C., & Ralston, L. (2020). *Australian home ownership: Past reflections, future directions*, No. 328. Melbourne: AHURI. http://www.ahuri.edu.au/research/final-reports/328, https://doi.org/10.18408/ahuri-5119801.

CHOICE, National Shelter & NATO (National Association of Tenants Organisations), (2017). *Unsettled: Life in Australia's private rental market*, Canberra.

Coates, B., & Chen, T. (2019). Retiree home ownership is about to plummet. Soon little more than half will own where they live, *The Conversation*, 19 April. https://theconversation.com/retiree-home-ownership-is-about-to-plummet-soon-little-more-than-half-will-own-where-they-live-115255.

Commission of Inquiry into Poverty. (1975a). *Poverty in Australia, first main report*, chair Professor R. F. Henderson. Canberra: AGPS (Australian Government Publishing Service).

Commission of Inquiry into Poverty. (1975b). *Law and poverty in Australia*, Second Main Report, Professor R. Sackville. Canberra: AGPS.

Commission of Inquiry into Poverty. (1975c). *Consumer views on welfare services and rented housing*, Research Report. Canberra: AGPS.

Commonwealth Housing Commission. (1944). *Final report: 25th August 1944.* Canberra: Ministry of Post-War Reconstruction.

Commonwealth Statistician. (1917). *Census of the commonwealth of Australia, Vol 1 statistician's report*, Census Bureau. Melbourne: Minister for State for Home and Territories, Melbourne.

CoreLogic. (2016). *Profile of the Australian residential property investor.* Irvine, CA: CoreLogic. https://soundproperty.com.au/wp-content/uploads/2018/01/CoreLogic-Investor-Report_June-2016.pdf.

Crook, T., & Kemp, P. (Eds.). (2014). *Private rental housing.* Cheltenham: Edward Elgar.

CURA (Centre for Urban Research and Action). (1979). *Landlords and lodgers: A study of rooming houses in Melbourne.* Fitzroy: Centre for Urban Research and Action.

Dalton, T., Pawson, H., & Hulse, K. (2015). *Rooming house futures: Governing for growth, fairness and transparency*, No. 245. Melbourne: AHURI. https://www.ahuri.edu.au/research/final-reports/245.

Daly, J., & Wood, D. (2016). *Hot property*. Melbourne: Grattan Institute. https://grattan.edu.au/report/hot-property/.

DSS (Department of Social Security). (1985). *Department of social security, annual report 1984–85*. Canberra: Australian Government.

DSS (Department of Social Services). (2019). *Department of social services annual report 2018–2019*. Canberra: Australian Government.

DSS (Department of Social Security). (1996, October). *Overview of the Australian private rental market*. Policy Research Paper No. 72. Canberra: Department of Social Security.

Ey, C. (2012). Supplementary allowance/assistance 1970 to 1985, Rent assistance from 1985 in *Social security payments for the unemployed, the sick and those in special circumstances, 1942 to 2012: A chronology*. Canberra: Parliament of Australia. https://www.aph.gov.au/About_Parliament/Parliamentary_Departments/Parliamentary_Library/pubs/BN/2012-2013/SSPaymentsUnemployment.

Fainstein, S. (2016). Financialisation and justice in the city: A commentary. *Urban Studies, 53*(7), 1503–1508.

Greenhalgh, E., Miller, A., Minnery, J., Gurran, N., Jacobs, N., & Phibbs, P. (2004). *Boarding houses and government supply side intervention*, No. 54. Melbourne: AHURI.

Harris, D. (1988). Not above politics: Housing reform in Melbourne 1910–1929. In R. Howe (Ed.), *New houses for old, fifty years of public housing in Victoria* (pp. 1–19). Mebourne: Ministry of Housing and Construction.

Hayward, D. (1996). The reluctant landlords? A history of public housing in Australia. *Urban Policy and Research, 14*(1), 5–35. http://doi.org/10.1080/08111149608551610.

Henderson, R. F., Harcourt, A., & Harper, R. J. A. (1970). *People in poverty, a Melbourne survey*. Melbourne: Cheshire for the Melbourne Institute of Applied Economic and Social Research.

Hulse, K. (2002). *Demand subsidies for private renters: A comparative review*. Final report. Australian Housing and Research Institute. http://www.ahuri.edu.au/pubs/finalreports.html.

Hulse, K., & Burke, T. (2015). Private rental housing in Australia: Political inertia and market change (Chapter 9). In R. Dufty-Jones & D. Rogers (Eds.), *Housing in 21st century Australia* (pp. 139–152). Farnham, UK: Ashgate.

Hulse, K., & McPherson, A. (2014). Exploring dual housing tenure status as a household response to demographic. *Social and Economic Change, Housing Studies, 29*(8), 1028–1044. https://doi.org/10.1080/02673037.2014.925097.

Hulse, K., Burke, T., Ralston, L., & Stone, W. (2012). *The Australian private rental sector: Changes and challenges*. Positioning Paper 149. Melbourne: AHURI.

Hulse, K., Reynolds, M., Nygaard, C., Parkinson, S., & Yates, J. (2019). *The supply of affordable private rental housing in Australian cities: Short-term and longer-term changes*, No. 323. Melbourne, AHURI. http://www.ahuri.edu.au/research/final-reports/323. https://doi.org/10.18408/ahuri5120101.

Jones, M. A. (1972). *Housing and poverty in Australia*. Melbourne: Melbourne University Press.

Kendig, H. (1979). *New life for old suburbs*. North Sydney: George Allen & Unwin.

Kewley, T. H. (1973). *Social security in Australia 1900–1972*. Sydney: Sydney University Press.

Kryger, T. (2009). *Home ownership in Australia data and trends*. Research Paper no. 21 2008–09. Canberra: Parliamentary Library. https://pdfs.semanticscholar.org/2782/d5fbd4ebdd0edd5020fc16cb0defb26ec2cc.pdf.

Logan, W. S. (1985). *The gentrification of inner Melbourne, a political geography of inner city housing*. St Lucia, Queensland: University of Queensland Press.

Madden, D., & Marcuse, P. (2016). *In defense of housing: The politics of crisis*. London and New York: Verso Books.

Martin, C., Hulse, K., & Pawson, H. with Hayden, A., Kofner, S., Schwartz, A., & Stephens, M. (2018). *The changing institutions of private rental housing: An international review*, No. 292. Melbourne: AHURI.

McCalman, J. (1993). *Journeyings: The biography of a middle-class generation 1920–1990*. Melbourne: Melbourne University Press.

McIntosh, G. (1997). *Reforming public housing, current issues, brief 31, 1996–97*. Canberra: Parliament of Australia, Parliamentary Library. https://www.aph.gov/About_Parliament/Parliamentary_Departments/Parliamentary_Library/pubs/BriefingBook45p/HousingAffordability.

Melbourne Institute. (2016). *Poverty lines: Australia, September quarter 2016*. Melbourne: Melbourne Institute of Applied Economic and Social Research, University of Melbourne.

Menzies, R. (1942). *The forgotten people*. Speech delivered 22 May 1942. http://www.liberals.net/theforgottenpeople.htm.

Morris, A. (2018) The financialisation of housing and the housing crisis in Sydney. *Housing Finance International, XXX11*(4), 63–69.

Mowbray, R. C. (1996). *The nature of contemporary landlordism in New South Wales: Implications for tenants' rights*. PhD thesis, Department of Urban and Regional Planning, Faculty of Architecture, University of Sydney (unpublished).

Neutze, M. (1977). *Urban development in Australia*. Sydney: George Allen & Unwin.

Neutze, M. (1978). *Australian urban policy*. Sydney: George Allen & Unwin.

O'Hanlon, S. (2002). 'All found' they used to call it': Genteel boarding houses in early twentieth-century Melbourne. *Urban History, 29*(2), 239–253.

Paris, C. (1984). *Affordable and available housing*, No. 117. Canberra: AIUS (Australian Institute of Urban Studies).

Paris, C. (1993). *Housing Australia*. South Melbourne: Macmillan Education (with A. Beer and W. Sanders).

Pawson, H., Milligan, V., & Yates, Y. (2020). *Housing policy in Australia*. Singapore: Palgrave Macmillan.

Power, E. (2017). Renting with pets: A pathway to housing insecurity? *Housing Studies, 32*(3), 336–360. http://doi.org/10.1080/02673037.2016.1210095.

Productivity Commission. (2017). *Introducing competition and informed user choice into human services: Reforms to human services*, Report No. 85, Canberra: Productivity Commission.

Productivity Commission. (2018). *Report on government services 2018, housing*. Canberra: Australian Government. https://www.pc.gov.au/research/ongoing/report-on-government-services/2017/housing-and-homelessness/housing/rogs-2017-volumeg-chapter18.pdf.

Productivity Commission. (2019). *Vulnerable private renters: Evidence and options*. Commission Research Paper, Canberra. https://www.pc.gov.au/research/completed/renters/private-renters.pdf.

Prosser, B., & Leeper, G. (1994, June). Housing affordability and changes to rent assistance. *Social Security Journal*, 58–61.

RBA (Reserve Bank of Australia). (2020). *Economic and financial statistics*. Indicator Lending Rates, Table F5. Sydney: RBA. https://www.rba.gov.au/statistics/tables/.

Ronald, R., & Kadi, J. (2018). The revival of private landlords in Britain's post-homeownership society. *New Political Economy, 23*(6), 786–803. https://doi.org/10.1080/13563467.2017.1401055.

Rowley, S., & James, A. (2018). *The private rental sector in Australia*. BCEC Research Report 18/18. Perth: Bankwest Curtin Economics Centre.

Simon, J., & Stone, T. (2017). *The property ladder after the financial crisis: The first step is a stretch but those who make it are doing oK*. Research Discussion Paper, RDP 2015-5. Sydney: RBA. https://www.rba.gov.au/publications/rdp/2017/pdf/rdp2017-05.pdf.

Stone, W., Burke, T., Hulse, K., & Ralston, L. (2013). *Long-term private rental in a changing Australian private rental sector* No. 209. Melbourne: AHURI.

Thomas, M., & Hall, A. (2016). *Housing affordability in Australia.* Canberra: Parliamentary Library. https://www.aph.gov.au/About_Parliament/Parliamentary_Departments/Parliamentary_Library/pubs/BriefingBook45p/HousingAffordability.

Thompson, R. (1986). *Sydney's flats, a social and political history*, PhD thesis, Macquarie University, Sydney (unpublished).

Tibbits, G. (1988). 'The enemy within our gates': Slum clearance and high-rise flats' (Chapter 6). In R. Howe (Ed.), *New houses for old. Fifty years of public housing in Victoria 1938–1988* (pp. 123–164). Melbourne: Ministry of Housing and Construction.

Vipond, J. (1987). Assisting private renters, social security review. Background Paper no. 18. Canberra: Department of Social Security.

Whitehead, C., Monk, S., Scanlon, K., Makkanen, S., & Tang, C. (2012). *The private rented sector in the new century—A comparative approach.* Cambridge: Cambridge Centre for Housing and Planning Research.

Whitten, W. (2020). *Historical Australian mortgage interest rates [updated].* Home Loan Finder. https://www.finder.com.au/historical-home-loan-interest-rates#svr.

Wilkins, R., & Vera-Toscano, E. (2019, 30 July). Over 50% of young Australian adults still live with their parents—And the numbers are climbing faster for women. *The Conversation.* https://theconversation.com/over-50-of-young-australian-adults-still-live-with-their-parents-and-the-numbers-are-climbing-faster-for-women-120587.

Wilkinson, J. (2005). *Affordable housing in NSW: Past to present.* Briefing paper 2005 No. 14. Sydney: NSW Parliamentary Library Research Service.

Wright, S. (2019, October 18). Sydney and Melbourne house prices will soon be growing at double-digit rates. *The Sydney Morning Herald.* https://www.smh.com.au/business/the-economy/sydney-and-melbourne-house-prices-will-soon-be-growing-at-double-digit-rates-20191018-p531z3.html.

Wulff, M., & Maher, C. (1998). Long-term renters in the Australian housing market. *Housing Studies, 13*(1), 83–98. https://doi.org/10.1080/02673039883506.

Wulff, M., Reynolds, M., Arunachalam, D., Hulse, K., & Yates, J. (2011). *Australia's private rental market: The supply of, and demand for, affordable dwellings.* No. 168, Melbourne, AHURI. https://www.ahuri.edu.au/research/final-reports/168.

Yates, J., Wulff, M., & Reynolds, M. (2004). *Changes in the supply of and need for low rent dwellings in the private rental market.* AHURI Final Report No. 61, Melbourne, Australian Housing and Urban Research Institute Limited. https://www.ahuri.edu.au/research/final-reports/61.

Chapter 2
Private Rental in Australia: A Lightly Regulated Sector

Abstract This chapter focuses on the body of regulation which sets the norms and expected behaviours involved in Australia's landlord-tenant relations. It opens by exploring the rationale for private rental regulation, especially in terms of the prevailing neo-liberal governance philosophy. Next, we present a national overview of tenancy regulation across Australia highlighting, where appropriate, particularly notable features of systems in specific jurisdictions. Drawing on this overview the chapter then discusses three key aspects of landlord-tenant relations, namely rent regulation, security of tenure and landlord repairing obligations. After briefly reviewing the distinct regulatory approaches that relate to boarding houses, we next summarise recent PRS regulatory reform debates and, in conclusion, reflect on the overall picture and future prospects for change in the balance of power between landlords and tenants.

Introduction

The experience of living as a private renter is highly dependent on the legal and administrative rules that govern landlord and tenant behaviour. These vary from country to country—and sometimes between cities or states within countries. What we are talking about here is the way that private rental housing is made available, the price (rent) that may be charged and the contractual terms on which a dwelling is occupied. All of these are influenced by government oversight or regulation, much of it embedded in law. So, although relatively modest in scale and reach by the standards of comparator countries (Martin et al., 2018), Australia's regulatory rules and practices importantly frame the workings of the PRS in this country and the experience of being a private renter.

In the last chapter, we saw that reforms to PRS regulation began in the late 1970s following Commission of Inquiry into Poverty and there were several subsequent waves of reform. To provide a basis for the remainder of the book, this chapter discusses the regulatory framework which effectively defines tenant rights in Australia. To underpin our overall contention that Australia's private landlords

A. Morris et al., *The Private Rental Sector in Australia*,
https://doi.org/10.1007/978-981-33-6672-5_2

operate within a system that is relatively favourable to their interests, the chapter compares Australia to countries in Europe and elsewhere.

As we also report below, the past decade has seen a notable upsurge of debate on PRS regulation in this country and in a number of other advanced economies; debates which have in some cases resulted in significant reforms.

Regulation sets the norms and expected behaviours of landlord-tenant relations. In Australia's housing history up to the late 1970s, such norms were adopted and adapted from English common law designed to cover land leases in agricultural societies rather than housing arrangements in a largely urban society (Bradbrook, 1975). Subsequently rental housing has been treated separately in specific state legislation. These Residential Tenancies Acts (RTAs) set out the legal and institutional framework for tenancy commencement, rent-setting, tenancy security and other tenant and landlord rights and responsibilities. While primarily relating to the mainstream PRS, the chapter also briefly discusses the special regulatory arrangements that typically apply to boarding houses[1] where the occupier lacks exclusive occupation rights to a self-contained dwelling.

As explained in Chapter 1, under Australia's constitution direct responsibility for land/housing management remains with the states and territories rather than the federal government. Since the 1970s state/territory RTAs have been re-conceptualised as consumer rights legislation (Bradbrook, 2003). Thus, the responsible government department is typically that charged with consumer protection. Over and above such consumer affairs departments, and as well as landlords and tenants themselves, other important stakeholders or institutions with an active role in sector regulation in most jurisdictions include tenants' unions that advocate for tenants' rights; property owners and landlords' associations that advocate for landlords' rights, and tribunals that rule on landlord-tenant disputes. When it comes to boarding houses, local councils are another important set of regulatory actors. They have the power to ensure the provision of safe and habitable conditions. All of these stakeholders have distinct interests and proposed changes to RTAs are typically hotly contested.

The remainder of the chapter is structured as follows. First, we discuss the rationale for private rental regulation, especially in terms of the neo-liberal governance philosophy that prevails in Australia. Next, we present a national overview of tenancy regulation which—albeit recognising the existence of eight sets of jurisdiction-specific rules—attempts to generalise as far as possible across the country. This is summarised in Table 2.1.

The next part of the chapter expands on and discusses each major aspect of the regulatory frameworks summarised in Table 2.1. Firstly, we discuss rent regulation; initially classifying the distinct forms this may assume, before noting the limited forms of such regulation that apply in contemporary Australia. Secondly, we consider tenants' rights on remaining in a rental dwelling (security of tenure). Thirdly, we discuss landlord obligations on property condition standards and the related issue of the administrative structures enabling tenants (or landlords) to seek redress when

[1] Referred to in Victoria as 'rooming houses'. For simplicity, the term boarding houses is used from this point onwards throughout the book.

Table 2.1 Mainstream PRS tenancy regulation in Australia: a national overview

		Generally	Of note
Access			
	Application forms and information	Unregulated	Provision in Victoria reforms to proscribe certain questions in applications for boarding house accommodation such as on the applicant's rental bond history
	Anti-discrimination	Discrimination in provision of accommodation on various grounds (race, sex, disability) prohibited under federal and state/territory anti-discrimination legislation	Some states prohibit discrimination against tenants with children in residential tenancies legislation
	Tenancy databases	Landlords and agents may use tenancy databases (not credit databases) to vet applications, obliged to notify tenant/applicant of listing	This applies only to recognised tenancy databases and does not include data collected and analysed by new business models using digital technology
	Costs at commencement	Limited to bond and rent in advance, both limited (mostly to four weeks and two weeks, respectively)	
	Bond protection	Landlords and agents required to lodge bonds with government agency (or statutory account: WA)	
	Information	Landlords and agents obliged to provide basic information statements about tenancy rights and responsibilities	Some matters specific to premises required to be disclosed (e.g. previous violence crime, bushfire zone, strata renewal: NSW)
Form of agreement			
	Prescribed forms	Prescribed standard forms and terms	Some contracting out allowed in WA, and NSW and Victoria (long fixed term agreements)

(continued)

Table 2.1 (continued)

	Written agreements	Landlord obliged to provide written copy, but oral agreements are still valid	
	Term	Lease agreements typically commence with a fixed term (usually 6 or 12 months—although this is not specified in law), and thereafter become periodic agreements if not terminated or subject to another fixed term	Initial fixed terms are not required, but as a matter of practice used almost everywhere. Queensland tenancies are often a succession of fixed terms; NSW tenancies more often commence with a fixed term then become periodic agreements (Choice et al., 2018)
Rent and other costs			
	Rent at commencement	Unregulated	
	Rent increases	Generally not permitted during fixed terms; otherwise permitted with written notice (mostly 2 months), not more than once in 6 (Qld, WA, NT) or 12 (NSW, SA, Tas, Vic, ACT) months	Victorian reform changing from up to twice a year to once a year
		Increases may be challenged if excessive relative to the market	
	Other costs	Limited to metred electricity, water, gas and septic tank pump out; not taxes or rates	
Tenants' privacy and quiet enjoyment			
	Quiet enjoyment	Prescribed term gives tenants right to quiet enjoyment	
		Prescribed terms prohibit tenants from causing nuisance, damage, or using premises for illegal purposes	
	Access by landlord	Various grounds with different notice periods and frequency (e.g. inspection, sale of property)	
	Pets	Additional term commonly proscribes pets without landlord's consent	

(continued)

Table 2.1 (continued)

Property conditions and repairs			
	Landlord's obligation	Prescribed terms oblige landlords to provide and maintain premises in reasonable repair	
		Some standards or facilities specified in NSW, Qld, Tas, Vic	Examples include smoke detectors (NSW), residual current detectors (Qld, WA)
	Emergency repairs	Tenants may carry out emergency repairs and seek recompense, subject to limits	Examples include electrical and plumbing problems
Tenancy termination			
	By tenants	Generally not permitted during fixed terms, except on prescribed grounds. At end of fixed term and in periodic agreement, termination permitted with and without grounds	
		Grounds include breach by landlord (mostly 2 weeks' notice), domestic violence-related circumstances	Also moving into social housing or aged care (NSW, Vic) Reforms re DV are recent
	By landlords	Generally not permitted during fixed terms, except on prescribed grounds. At end of fixed term and in periodic agreement, termination permitted with and without grounds (except Tas and Vic)	Tas: termination of periodic agreement without grounds not permitted Vic, termination without grounds now not permitted, except at end of first fixed term
		No-grounds notice periods range from 42 days (NT) to 26 weeks (ACT)	
		Grounds include breach by tenant (mostly 2 weeks' notice), sale of premises and landlord and/or family moving into the premises	Vic has a more comprehensive set of prescribed grounds, including change of use and landlord to use premises for own housing

(continued)

Table 2.1 (continued)

	By third parties	Mortgagees may take termination and possession proceedings where landlord is in default	SA and NT provide for termination proceedings by third parties (including neighbours)
Dispute resolution			
	Dispute resolution forums	Disputes and termination proceedings determined by Civil and Administrative Tribunals (except Tas and WA); cheaper and less formal than courts	Previous specialist residential tenancy tribunals have been rolled into 'super' tribunals (CATs) Tas and WA use Magistrates Courts
	Retaliation	Tribunal may decline to terminate a tenancy where landlord's proceedings are retaliation for assertion of tenancy rights	NT (alone) proscribes retaliation against tenants who join tenant associations

Sources Martin et al. (2018, 2021). The authors are indebted to Dr. Chris Martin for assembling this table. *Note* Abbreviations used NT is Northern Territories, Tas is Tasmania, Vic is Victoria, SA is South Australia, WA is West Australia, NSW is New South Wales, ACT is Australian Capital territory

dwelling condition or other matters are in dispute. Next, given the specific rules that apply to boarding houses, we briefly review the regulatory approaches that generally relate to that context. In the chapter's penultimate section we summarise recent PRS regulatory reform debates, and in conclusion we reflect on the overall picture and future prospects for change in the balance of power between landlords and tenants.

Regulatory Context and Rationale

The extent and form of private rental regulation in Australia is framed within a broader national governance setting. Largely in keeping with fellow Anglosphere nations, the modus operandi of Australian governments is strongly influenced by the neo-liberal paradigm dominant since the 1980s.

Although its precise meaning is contested, neo-liberalism broadly describes a governance approach that prioritises deregulation and the optimal use of resources as paramount, maintains a stated commitment to consumer sovereignty and places faith in the market and the unfettered exercise of user choice as a means of maximising efficient outcomes (Le Grand et al., 2008; Whitehead, 2012). Its adherents see government actions that constrain or shape the operation of market processes—e.g. through administratively-set prices for goods or services—as interventions liable to distort market outcomes in a problematic way. Proponents argue that such rules will impair market efficiency. They also conflict with sometimes associated libertarian beliefs on property ownership rights, viz the rights to acquire, hold, determine occupancy and use, and to dispose of residential assets. It should be noted, however, that the cultural dominance of property rights in Australia predates neoliberalism.

Neo-liberal thinking, as applied to the domain of housing since the 1980s, regards government intervention as usually undesirable. Unlike spaces for major state involvement acknowledged as legitimate—e.g. provision of health or education services—housing is considered a domain where markets generally function effectively to the benefit of all. In reality, active state facilitation and involvement is inherent to the effective operation of markets, at the least via maintenance of orderly legal and regulatory frameworks such as a reliable land title system, law on contracts and consumer protection, regulation on financing and property transactions. These perspectives are just as true when it comes to private rental housing markets as in relation to the private provision of other goods and services.

Neo-liberal thinking nevertheless recognises the concept of 'market failure' and accepts that the correction of such failure can be a legitimate justification for government intervention—in the housing domain, just as in other services and sectors (Le Grand et al., 2008; Whitehead, 2012).

In the broadest terms, market failure describes any situation where the production, consumption and investment choices of individuals do not result in outcomes that maximise collective benefit. This may arise in market conditions that infringe assumptions inherent to the model of so-called perfect competition. Two such assumptions are of particular relevance here. Firstly, that there are 'many buyers and sellers' and implicitly, therefore, power is equally held by both sets of parties. And, secondly, that all market players possess perfect information about product quality and alternatives within that market and can make rational decisions guided by their self-interest.

When it comes to rental housing transactions, however, any expectation that all players have equal power and are perfectly informed is fallacious. Thus, if a rental property 'acquires the status of a home for a tenant and the tenant becomes attached to his [sic] home, the landlord acquires a monopolistic power to raise the rent. Indeed, the tenant must incur high financial and emotional costs to move and thus avoid the rent increase' (Haffner et al., 2018, p. 219). This is all the more challenging for low income renters who have little or no market power enabling them to shop around for a better housing deal. On this basis, as contended by Haffner et al. (2018), far from distorting or damaging market dynamics, regulation of rental housing can 'improve economic efficiency'. From this perspective, therefore, tenant protection via rent regulation may be portrayed as necessary to counteract a market-distorting power imbalance.

While neo-liberal ideas continue to pervade governance approaches globally, the degree of dominance and application of these ideas varies between countries—or groups of countries. In particular, in some of the Northern European nations with which Australia is often compared when it comes to private rental regulation, social democratic and/or corporatist traditions continue to exercise significant influence over policymaking and institutional structures, even if these conventions have been recently eroded. Thus, the regulation of private rental markets in nations such as

Denmark, the Netherlands and Germany is conducted against a distinctly different cultural and governance backdrop to that prevailing in Australia, New Zealand, the UK, Canada and the USA (Crook and Kemp, 2014).

At the same time, the post-GFC period has seen a significant shift in European and UK housing policymaker thinking as regards PRS regulation (Haffner et al., 2018; Robertson & Young, 2018; Whitehead & Williams, 2018). According to Haffner and colleagues (2018, p. 19), a largely unqualified belief in minimally regulated markets, has given way to a faith in 'smart regulation' aimed at reducing the risk of 'market failures caused by information asymmetry, politically biased tenure policy, and the lack of the right incentives'. As cited here, smart regulation is defined as actions that 'proactively [strive] … to create the economic and political conditions of an efficient market system' (ibid.). Whether such observations are reflected in recent Australian policy debates is a question we revisit later in this chapter.

Tenancy Regulation in Australia: A National Overview

The overall approach to PRS oversight remains fundamentally similar across Australia, notwithstanding that each of Australia's eight states and territories has its own specific rules and institutional frameworks. As noted above, these are primarily embodied in each jurisdiction's RTA. With only limited exceptions, all such frameworks embody deeply-embedded assumptions about the primacy of property rights. Consistent with these orientations, PRS regulation to protect tenants rights is relatively weak by the standards of many other advanced economies (Blunden & Martin, 2003; National Shelter & NATO, 2010).

As a summary of the key features of tenancy regulation that currently prevail across Australia, Table 2.1 provides a basis for the remainder of this chapter. Specific aspects of the table are further discussed in subsequent sections. It should be noted that private rental housing is also subject to regulation of other kinds, including anti-discrimination legislation (Hulse et al., 2011).

Rent Regulation

As discussed in Chapter 1, significant restrictions on permissible rents were widely imposed in Australia in the early post-World War 2 era, as in many other developed nations. Similarly, once again in keeping with international trends, succeeding decades saw such controls largely dismantled in this country (see below). As noted above, however, at least in Europe the post-GFC era has seen some revival of interest in private rental regulation triggered by sector expansion and growing tenant stress in some cities with pressured housing markets. As further discussed below, in some countries this has included the reappearance of statutory rent restrictions.

The conventional wisdom on restricting the price of rental housing at below its market level is that this is always undesirable because it is likely to disincentivise new provision, as well as leading to poorly-maintained dwellings and landlords exiting the market. This view has been largely unchallenged in Australia. Thus, the orthodox position is that while rent control 'can benefit those fortunate enough to occupy a rent-controlled property', such rules 'ultimately reduce the supply and quality of rental housing and, perversely, may even make it more difficult for a low-income household to secure a lease' (Productivity Commission, 2019, p. 12).

However, while it has been noted that 'opposition to rent control is something like an oath of office for the [Economics] profession' (Metcalf, 2018, p. 66), there is an in principle economic rationale for some form of rent regulation within a market economy context, as prevails in Australia. Considering the typically 'sticky' response of housing supply to rising demand for rental property, it is argued that such tenant protection may be theoretically justified. Under such conditions 'rents rise often well above the longer-term costs of provision' and, as a result, landlords may consequently reap 'excess profits' (Whitehead & Williams, 2018, p. 8). On this basis, Arnott (1995) argued the case for rent regulation as a means of enhancing (rather than distorting) PRS market equilibrium.

Nevertheless, 'rent control' comes in a number of distinctly different forms—and many of the arguments over rent regulation's pros and cons are highly dependent on the type of restriction under consideration. We therefore need to explore this in greater depth.

Conventionally, a rent regulation distinction is made between the restriction of *rent levels* (sometimes termed 'hard rent control') and the limitation of *rent increases* ('soft rent control'). Thus, under this typology:

- First generation controls place limits on all rent levels
- Second generation controls limit rent increases within and between tenancies
- Third generation controls limit rent increases within tenancies only.

(Arnott, 1995, p. 2003).
The rent controls that applied in Australia and comparator countries in the early post-war period were first generation restrictions—government-imposed below-market maxima for properties of particular types in particular areas. Restrictions of this sort are vulnerable to the criticism that—because they suppress gross rental yields (the ratio of rents to property values)—they discourage landlords from investing in additional properties or properly maintaining existing rental homes. Perhaps more importantly, they may encourage landlords to transfer rental properties to other uses—e.g. sale for owner occupation or re-purposing boarding houses for other uses as discussed in Chapter 1.

Since the 1970s, private landlords in Australia have been required to observe only 'light touch' third generation restrictions—that is, rules protecting existing tenants from the risk that their reluctance or inability to move might be exploited via unjustifiably large rent increases relative to the market. Such rules incorporate provision for tenants to dispute increases considered 'unreasonable' on this basis, with adjudication typically provided by a tenancy tribunal (see below). Very similar light touch rent regulation operates in England and Wales, among other countries.

Similarly classifiable as third generation regulation, but providing somewhat stronger protection in 'hot' housing markets (where market rents may be rising ahead of other prices), are rules which limit within-tenancy increases to a defined benchmark such as the general rate of inflation. New measures of this kind—or provision for them—have been recently introduced in several European countries including Ireland and Scotland (Robertson and Young, 2018). Nonetheless, critics report that landlords in booming European cities subject to such rules have been able to 'largely ignore them' because tenants, keen to secure or retain a tenancy, opt not to enforce their newly gained rights (Robertson and Young, 14).

Only in a few developed countries (or a few cities within such nations) do first—or even second—generation rules remain in place (Martin et al., 2018). However, a number of European and North American cities have recently heard strident calls for the return of hard rent control—activism that has, in some instances, triggered significant action. In Berlin, for example, rising popular discontent triggered by rent inflation led to the 2019 announcement of a five-year rent freeze across the city (Blackman, 2019). Meanwhile, New York State moved in 2019 to 'abolish rules that let building owners deregulate apartments, clos[ing] a series of loopholes that permit them to raise rents and allow[ing] some tenant protections to expand statewide' (Ferre Sadurni et al., 2019).

Within the context of an international comparative study, Martin et al. (2018) suggested that stronger forms of third generation rent regulation could be reasonably considered for Australia. Beyond this agitation for rent control has remained extremely rare in Australia over the last five decades. Rather, enhancement of tenant security has tended to be much more of a priority for rental reform campaigners.

Security of Tenure

In housing policy parlance, security of tenure is generally understood as a legal arrangement in which a tenant enjoys an indefinite right to occupy their home, subject only to proven breaches of their lease agreement or other provisions, e.g. landlord selling the property or wanting to occupy the property that provide grounds for termination action by their landlord. For any individual renter, their security of tenure is the degree to which this state of affairs exists; although, as discussed in Chapter 7, there are a range of factors that may contribute to a tenant's sense of security or insecurity.

Private landlords in Australia are not entirely free to summarily end tenancies at will. Nevertheless, by comparison with their situation in many comparator nations, private renters lack legal security. This reflects the country's market liberal social and economic tradition, and the cultural weight attached to property ownership which influences housing policy more broadly (Pawson et al., 2020). Landlord practice is usually to rent dwellings on a six or 12-month fixed-term basis, with the tenant often offered a further fixed-term of similar duration at expiry. Alternatively, the agreement reverts to a periodic tenancy that can be terminated by either party upon service of required notice.

For leases that have reverted to periodic status, landlords are generally free to recover possession of the dwelling. Until recent changes in Victoria (see below), it was only in Tasmania (for periodic tenancies) that an owner needed to justify this demand in terms of defined 'legitimate grounds' for termination. To put this another way, 'no grounds evictions' have remained generally allowable in law. Although they must respect a legally-defined notice period when seeking to end a tenancy, a landlord is under no obligation to specify a legally-sanctioned reason.

As specified in Australian state/territory law, once the lease/written agreement ends, tenancy termination notice periods vary across jurisdictions (see Table 2.1). The notice period depends on the reason for the repossession, and whether the existing arrangement is an expiring fixed-term tenancy or periodic arrangement. Thus, where relating to a property being repossessed for sale and occupied under a periodic contract, the specified notice period is generally 30–60 days. A 'no grounds' repossession (as remains legally allowable in most jurisdictions) may require the landlord to give the tenant written notice of between 42 days (NT) and 26 weeks (ACT)—see Table 2.1.

Minimum tenancy-end notice periods in Australia tend to be shorter than internationally (Productivity Commission, 2019). Short notice periods can be extremely problematic for tenants. In a tight rental market finding alternative accommodation in a short period of time can be difficult and stressful (see Chapters 4 and 7). This is especially so for low-income households. Also, longer notice periods could enhance tenant welfare, partly on the basis that they would increase tenants' bargaining power, as they will be placed under less pressure by a landlord decision to end a tenancy if they have longer to seek alternatives. In some cases, due to personal circumstances, it is in the tenant's interest to be able to give a short notice period if their circumstances have changed.

PRS Security of Tenure in Australia Compared to Other Countries

More broadly, as indicated in Table 2.2, private tenants in Australia typically have more limited security of tenure than in some comparator countries. While not dissimilar from frameworks in New Zealand and England and Wales, as well as parts of the USA, Australian state/territory regimes differ from those in Canada (where no grounds terminations are often proscribed), but more fundamentally from those of most Northern European countries where open-ended tenancies are the norm.

To highlight a contrasting security of tenure regime in more detail, Box 2.1 illustrates the very limited circumstances in which tenancies can be ended in Germany where tenants generally enjoy open-ended security of tenure. Although this is a notable feature of the German housing system we are not wanting to imply here that

Table 2.2 Security of tenure: Australasia, Europe, North America (selected countries)

Country	Fixed term and periodic tenancies	Grounds for termination by landlord
Austria	Multi-dwelling tenancies open-ended; single dwellings minimum 3-year fixed term	Prescribed grounds only
Australia	Short (6–12 months), fixed-term and periodic tenancies	No-grounds termination allowed (except in Tasmania and Victoria)
Belgium	3-year and 9-year fixed terms	Termination at end of fixed term allowed
Canada	Mostly short (6–12 months), fixed-term and periodic tenancies	Mostly prescribed grounds only; some allow termination at end of fixed term
Germany	Tenancies typically open-ended	Prescribed grounds only
Ireland	Short fixed-term and periodic tenancies	Prescribed 6-year cycle with lesser restrictions on termination in initial 6 months, then prescribed grounds only
New Zealand	Short (6–12 months), fixed-term and periodic tenancies	No-grounds termination allowed
Sweden	Tenancies typically open-ended	Prescribed grounds only
Spain	3-year fixed terms with some provision for early termination	Termination at end of and, in limited circumstances during, fixed term
The Netherlands	Tenancies typically open-ended	Prescribed grounds only
United Kingdom	Short (6–12 months), fixed-term and periodic tenancies	No-grounds termination allowed (England and Wales); prescribed grounds only (Scotland)
United States	Short fixed-term and periodic tenancies	Varies by state and municipality: termination without grounds generally allowed; prescribed grounds only in a few large cities

Source Martin et al. (2018); Hulse et al. (2011)

housing policy in that country is in all important respects superior to other comparable nations. It is nevertheless worth emphasising that, since strong tenant protection co-exists with one of the largest private rental sectors in Europe, the German case argues against any simplistic claim that privileging tenant interests is fundamentally incompatible with mass private rental provision (Whitehead et al., 2012).

Box 2.1: Tenancy security in Germany

Private tenants in Germany generally enjoy strong security of tenure (see Kofner, 2018). This is provided through regulating the termination grounds and notice periods that must be observed by landlords, rather than through fixed term tenancies. Open-ended rental agreements are the norm. Such a contract may be terminated only where there is a 'legitimate interest', specifically:

- The tenant's wilful or negligent substantial breach of contract
- 'Hindrance to economic exploitation' (in practice, demolition of the premises)
- Property needed as a residence for the landlord or a family member
- Conversion of adjoining rooms to living space.

Under the 'hindrance to economic exploitation' ground, a landlord's decision to demolish must be 'reasonable and comprehensible'. The need to replace the building to remedy fundamentally poor property condition or obsolescence may be acceptable arguments for ending a tenancy in these circumstances. In practice, landlord termination is most commonly invoked on the 'personal need' ground.

Substantial notice periods (three months minimum) are also mandatory; notice periods are extended for tenancies of longer existing duration. There is also provision for a tenant to challenge tenancy termination where this would cause them 'undue hardship'—a claim that will be legally adjudicated. In any event evictions can be undertaken only where endorsed by a court order.

Strong security of tenure enjoyed by Germany's tenants has remained largely unchanged for decades and is little debated. 'These rules seem to be so deeply ingrained that it would be tantamount to political suicide to touch them' (Kofner, 2014, p. 42).

Property Condition, Maintenance and the Resolution of Landlord-Tenant Disputes

While there are minor technical differences from state to state, tenants across Australia face generally similar arrangements when it comes to the rules for rental property condition and maintenance standards landlords must observe. Likewise, the means for resolving landlord-tenant disputes on these and other matters are also based on a similar model in all eight jurisdictions. The key instrument here is typically the relevant state/territory Residential Tenancies Act (RTA).

As it is usually phrased in the prevailing state/territory RTA, a landlord must ensure that, at the point of letting, a dwelling is rented out 'in a reasonable state of repair'. It must also be 'reasonably clean' and 'fit for habitation'. Similarly, during the tenancy, a landlord must maintain the home in a 'reasonable state of repair'. Being embedded within standard tenancy contracts, such expectations form a binding contractual commitment. However, although some RTAs include practical examples of what these terms could mean in practice, these are generally presented as illustrative only.[2] There is, therefore, a degree of subjectivity in terms of what might be considered 'reasonable'.[3]

[2]For example, under NSW RTA amendments in force from 2020, more specific guidance has been included on "fitness for habitation"—see S52(1)(A).

[3]Although the NSW RTA 2010 provides some guidance in stating that "reasonable standard of repair" means "having regard to the age of, rent payable for, and prospective life of the premises" (S63(2)). The requirement for smoke alarms is a notable exception to the general rule that RTAs stand back from explicitly defining "reasonable state of repair".

In the spirit of the Australian 'consumer rights' model of PRS regulation (Bradbrook, 2003), tenants with property condition complaints are expected to assert such rights through a designated official tribunal. In doing so, they are making the case that the landlord has breached the terms of tenancy contract. In NSW the adjudicating body is the NSW Civil and Administrative Tribunal (NCAT). The Victorian Civil and Administrative Tribunal (VCAT) is that state's equivalent entity. Thus, under the consumer rights approach, responsibility for identifying and challenging landlord non-compliance with legal expectations rests with the tenant—rather than with any other body such as the local council.

In Victoria, in 2018–19, there were 52,412 applications to VCAT Residential Tenancies Division of which 6,693 were made by tenants/residents. Private landlords (typically represented by real estate agents) accounted for (35,803), with the remainder lodged by the Victorian Government (as public housing provider) or others (VCAT, 2019). Such disputes tend to relate to rent arrears, landlord claims for property re-possession, and tenant complaints on unreturned bonds.

A Tribunal decision in favour of a tenant complaint on disrepair may result in an order for a rent reduction—on the basis that such a landlord failure 'amounts to a withdrawal of goods, services and facilities provided' (Martin, 2012, p. 50). In some instances, a compensation payment may result.

Under recently introduced procedures in NSW, it has been made possible for tenants to take a landlord complaint direct to the state government's Fair Trading Department so as to avoid the formality of a tribunal application. How this will work in practice has yet to be seen.

The most important shortcoming of the arrangements described above is their limited utility within a context where a tenant's security of tenure remains weak. Here we are referring to fact that, as discussed earlier, in most parts of Australia it remains possible for a landlord to bring a periodic tenancy to an end without the need to specify termination grounds. In these circumstances, fear of retaliatory eviction is likely to mean that many tenants with concerns about landlord behaviour—including failure to commission requested repairs—will be reluctant to assert their rights via the formal channels available.

Regulating Boarding Houses

Beyond what is often conceptualised as the 'mainstream' private rental market is a diverse portfolio often referred to as 'marginal rental' housing where occupancy standards are markedly lower and rents cheaper than mainstream market norms (Goodman et al., 2013). This includes caravan parks and informal housing such as 'beds in sheds' or sleep outs and garages. By its very nature, such accommodation is below the radar of regulation and, hence, not discussed in this chapter.

Perhaps the most important component of marginal rental housing involves accommodation where residents rent individual rooms and share facilities such as kitchens and bathrooms. Such buildings are termed 'rooming houses' (Victoria) or 'boarding houses' (NSW and elsewhere). Residents have different legal rights from mainstream PRS tenants. Also, the buildings are subject to specific legal and regulatory codes, reflecting associated health and safety hazards (Dalton et al., 2015a).

According to the official census definition, people occupying boarding houses in 2016 numbered some 17,500—a 17% increase over the 2011 total (Pawson et al., 2018). In 2014, the number of buildings officially registered as such in New South Wales and Victoria totalled 774 and 1,131, respectively (Pawson et al., 2015; Dalton et al., 2015b). At the same time, sector experts believe that these numbers significantly understate the number of premises that effectively act as rooming/boarding house accommodation in these two states.

Rooming/boarding houses are of particular regulatory concern for several reasons. First, as the cheapest and most basic form of rental housing they tend to act as last resort accommodation for vulnerable individuals excluded from mainstream accommodation by their low income and/or other factors such as being a recently-released ex-offender. Second, shared occupancy conditions can accentuate safety risks hazards, especially fire. Third, they are often high turnover establishments, which may make them more liable to be a source of local disturbance.

Traditionally, rooming/boarding house residents have enjoyed fewer tenancy rights than mainstream PRS tenants. This derives from the formal legal distinction between 'tenancy'—where the resident enjoys exclusive occupancy—and 'lodging'—where this is not the case. Under 2012 NSW boarding house reforms residents were afforded formal occupancy rights, including the right to reasonable written notice of eviction—consistent with the agreed terms of the resident's occupancy agreement. Disputes with proprietors could now be lodged with the NSW Civil and Administrative Tribunal (NCAT). Rooming house residents in Victoria enjoy a certain amount of security in relation to the risk of being displaced by a building's sale or renovation; if asked to leave in these circumstances, they must be provided with 60 days written notice.

Local councils are important stakeholders in the regulation of rooming/boarding houses. In both NSW and Victoria, establishment owners must register with the relevant council. Councils are responsible for building inspection and other oversight to ensure that prescribed safety standards are maintained.

Reforming Private Rental Regulation

As discussed in Chapter 1, a major wave of PRS regulatory reform was triggered by a scathing report from the Commission of Inquiry into Poverty in 1975 (Braybrook, 1975). Since then there have been further reform moves affecting matters such as bond and rent in advance payments and repair and maintenance rights and responsibilities. Central to recent rental reform campaigns in Australia has been the demand to outlaw 'no grounds evictions'. A landlord's ability to end a tenancy at will (except while a fixed term remains in force) is problematic because, in the sober language of the

Productivity Commission (a federal government research report) (2019, p. 120), the availability of this option

> increases the bargaining power of landlords…and decreases that of tenants. [Moreover] landlords' incentives to carry out obligations, such as repairs and maintenance, decrease when no grounds evictions are available, since this provides them with an avenue to terminate leases in the event of a dispute.

Emulating a number of other countries included in Table 2.2, the Victorian Government announced in 2018 that no grounds evictions would be outlawed under a new reform package eventually implemented in 2021. Henceforward, as in countries such as Germany, tenancies may be ended by landlords only where the tenant has breached the terms of tenancy (e.g. through rent arrears), where the property is needed for the landlord's own occupation or where it is to be renovated or sold.

Although the proscription of no grounds evictions was considered in the NSW State Parliament in 2019, the State Government opted against any change on the basis that the status quo (freedom to end a tenancy without needing to specify a reason) could be desirable for landlords wishing to 'maintain their privacy and not disclose their personal affairs to tenants…' (Productivity Commission, 2019, p. 120). At the time of writing the Queensland Government was considering a package of possible changes to rental laws including no grounds eviction.

The outlawing of no grounds evictions—as carried through in Victoria—certainly strengthens tenants' security of tenure. However, it falls short of offering open-ended tenure security, most particularly because the 'specified grounds' on which a landlord may legitimately end a tenancy include property sale. In its advocacy for 'an end to no cause evictions' the UK lobby group, *Generation Rent*, argues that intent to sell should be excluded from the acceptable reasons for ending a tenancy. This implies that a landlord's rights in this eventuality would be limited to sale—with sitting tenant in situ—to another landlord. However, despite the fact that landlord to landlord sales may be quite common in Australia (Pawson & Martin, 2020) calls for such reform have yet to be voiced here.

In any consideration of possible reforms to landlord-tenant law, a crucial reality to be kept in mind is the indivisibility of rents from tenancy security. That is, 'rents cannot be regulated effectively if tenancies can be readily terminated and legal security is ineffective if rents can be increased without restriction' (Martin et al., 2018, p. 52). In other words, any effort to control or limit the rent payable within a tenancy cannot work unless there are also controls to restrict the landlord's ability to end that tenancy—and, thereby, re-let the dwelling at a higher charge. Equally, if the policy priority is to provide a measure of tenant security by limiting the landlord's right to end a tenancy, some limits on rent increases are also necessary so that this policy aim cannot be frustrated by unreasonable rent increases aimed at securing the tenant's 'voluntary' departure.

Other reform demands voiced in recent Australian tenants' rights campaigns have included enforcement of minimum property standards and a default tenant right to pet ownership (Bale, 2018). Thus, while security of tenure considerations are central, the range of matters at issue also encompasses other aspects of a tenant's conditions of occupancy. In conceptualising this more holistic view of PRS 'fitness for purpose' from a tenant perspective, the notion of 'secure occupancy' has been developed (Hulse & Milligan, 2014). This is further discussed in Chapter 7.

Conclusions

Private rental housing in Australia is lightly regulated by international standards. Restrictions on the rent that may be charged and the circumstances in which tenancies may be ended are modest as compared with at least some comparator countries. It is a set of arrangements that have been 'heavily weighted in favour of landlords and against the interests of tenants' (Burke, 2012, p. 39). However, as in Europe and North America, the past decade has seen growing calls for a re-balancing of landlord and tenant rights—especially when it comes to enhancing tenant security. The significant reforms coming into effect in Victoria in 2021 and the strong pressures for reform in other jurisdictions, suggest that long-established policy settings that have given landlords inordinate power are beginning to shift in a significant way. There is little doubt that the scrapping of no grounds eviction, longer notice periods and more significant limitations on rent increases would augment tenant welfare and enhance the attractiveness of private renting in Australia.

References

Arnott, R. (1995). Time for revisionism on rent control? *Journal of Economic Perspectives, 9*(1), 99–120.

Arnott, R. (2003). *Swedish economic policy review* (Vol. 10, pp. 89–121). Stockholm: Ministry of Finance.

Bale, B. (2018, November 1). Ideas of home and ownership in Australia might explain the neglect of renters' rights. *The Conversation*. https://theconversation.com/ideas-of-home-and-ownership-in-australia-might-explain-the-neglect-of-renters-rights-104849.

Blackman, A. (2019, October 21). Berlin freezes rents in landmark plan to tackle cost spiral. *Bloomberg*. https://www.bloomberg.com/news/articles/2019-10-18/berlin-government-reaches-deal-to-freeze-rents-for-5-years.

Blunden, H., & Martin, C. (2003). *Leaking roofs: Australian tenancy law. A report by the National Association of Tenant Organisation*. Sydney: Tenants' Union of New South Wales.

Bradbrook, A. J. (1975). *Poverty and the residential landlord-tenant relationship*. Canberra: Australian Government Publishing Service (AGPS).

Bradbrook, A. J. (2003). Rented housing law: Past, present and future. *Flinders Journal of Law Reform, 7*(1), 1–14.

Burke, T. (2012). The Australian residential housing market: Institutions and actors. In R. Tomlinson (Ed.), *Australia's Unintended Cities*. Melbourne: CSIRO.

Choice, National Shelter and the National Association of Tenant Organizations. (2018). *Disrupted: The consumer experience of renting in Australia*. Marrickville, NSW: Choice. https://www.choice.com.au/-/media/cb55695ea54d4f928802aa78b1b9c60a.ashx?la=en.

Crook, T., & Kemp, P. A. (Eds.). (2014). *Private rental housing: Comparative perspectives*. Cheltenham: Edward Elgar.

Dalton, T., Pawson, H., & Hulse, K. (2015a). *Rooming house futures: Governing for growth, fairness and transparency*, No. 245. Melbourne: AHURI.

Dalton, T., Hulse, K., & Pawson, H. (2015b). *Rooming house futures: Governing for growth, transparency and fairness—Victorian Discussion Paper*. Melbourne: AHURI.

Ferré-Sadurní, L., McKinley, J., & Wang, V. (2019, June 11). Landmark deal reached on rent protections for tenants in N.Y. *New York Times*. https://www.nytimes.com/2019/06/11/rent-protection-regulation.html.

Goodman, R., Nelson, A., Dalton, T., Cigdem, M., Gabriel, M., & Jacobs, K. (2013). *The experience of marginal rental housing in Australia*, No. 210. Melbourne: AHURI.

Haffner, M., Hegedüs, J., & Knorr-Siedow, T. (2018). The private rental sector in Western Europe. In J. Hegedűs, M. Lux, & V. Horváth (Eds.), *Private rental housing in transition countries: An alternative to owner occupation?* London: Palgrave.

Hulse, K. Milligan, V., & Easthope, H. (2011). *Secure occupancy in rental housing: Conceptual foundations and comparative perspectives*, No. 170. Melbourne: AHURI.

Hulse, K., & Milligan, V. (2014). Secure occupancy: A new framework for analysing security in rental housing. *Housing Studies, 29*(5), 638–656.

Le Grand, J., Propper, C., & Smith, S. (2008). *The economics of social problems* (4th ed.). Basingstoke: Palgrave Macmillan.

Kofner, S. (2014). The German housing system: Fundamentally resilient? *Journal of Housing and the Built Environment, 29*(2), 255–275.

Kofner, S. (2018). Appendix 1: Private rental housing in Germany. In C. Martin, K. Hulse, & H. Pawson (Eds.), *The changing institutions of private rental housing: An international review*, No. 292. Melbourne: AHURI.

Martin, C. (2012). *Tenants' rights manual*. Sydney: Federation Press.

Martin, C. (2021). Australia's incipient eviction crisis: No going back. *Alternative Law Journal*. https://doi.org/10.1177/1037969X21990940.

Martin, C., Hulse, K., & Pawson, H. (2018). *The changing institutions of private rental housing: An international review*, No. 292. Melbourne: AHURI.

Metcalf, G. (2018). Sand castles before the tide? Affordable housing in expensive cities. *Journal of Economic Perspectives, 32*(1), 59–80.

National Shelter & NATO. (2010). *A better lease on life: Improving Australian tenancy law*. Canberra: National Shelter.

Pawson, H., Dalton, T., & Hulse, K. (2015). *Rooming house futures: Governing for growth, transparency and fairness—New South Wales Discussion Paper*. Melbourne: AHURI.

Pawson, H., Parsell, C., Saunders, P., Hill, P., & Liu, E. (2018). *Australian homelessness monitor 2018*. Melbourne: Launch Housing.

Pawson, H., & Martin, C. (2020). Rental property investment in disadvantaged areas: The means and motivations of Western Sydney's new landlords. *Housing Studies*—Online first. https://doi.org/10.1080/02673037.2019.1709806.

Pawson, H., Milligan, V., & Yates, J. (2020). *Housing policy in Australia: A case for system reform*. Singapore: Palgrave.

Productivity Commission (2019). *Vulnerable private renters: Evidence and options*. Canberra: Australian Government.

Robertson, D., & Young, G. (2018). *An evaluation of rent regulation measures within Scotland's private rented sector*. Edinburgh: Shelter Scotland.

VCAT (Victoria Civil and Administrative Claims Tribunal). (2019). *Annual Report 2018–19*. Melbourne: VCAT. https://www.vcat.vic.gov.au/sites/default/files/resources/annual-report-2018-19.PDF. Accessed 26 Jan 2020.

Whitehead, C. (2012). The neo-liberal legacy to housing research. In D. Clapham, W. A. V. Clark, & K. Gibb, (Eds.), *The sage handbook of housing studies*. London: Sage.

Whitehead, C., Monk, S., Scanlon, K., Markkanen, S., & Tang, C. (2012). *The private rented sector in the new century: A comparative approach.* London: LSE.
Whitehead, C., & Williams, P. (2018). *Assessing the evidence on rent control: An international perspective.* Manchester: Residential Landlords Association.

Chapter 3
Private Rental Property Ownership

Abstract Research on Australia's private rental sector (PRS) has tended to focus on the demand side of the market. However, to properly comprehend how the sector functions an understanding of the landlord cohort, their motivations and behaviour, is also essential. This chapter therefore concentrates on the individuals and entities who provide private rental housing in Australia, on the sector's evolving ownership structure, and on the market conditions and policy settings that have influenced this. To help frame and explain the changing nature and scale of private rental housing investment the chapter reviews key influencing developments in global financial markets, as well as Australia's tax settings and regulatory levers that contribute towards shaping landlord behaviours. The chapter's prime focus is the nation's 2.2 million small-scale rental property owners who provide the vast bulk of Australia's mainstream PRS housing stock. However, recognising the possibility that it might come to form a significant sector component in future, institutionally-financed and owned 'build to rent' housing is also discussed.

Introduction

Research on Australia's private rental sector (PRS) has tended to focus on the demand side of the market rather than its supply dimension. As discussed in Chap. 1, studies have typically concentrated on tenants' conditions of occupancy (e.g. affordability and tenure security), and on landlord-tenant relations (see Chap. 2). Investigation of private rental housing supply or provision—PRS properties and their ownership—has been generally thinner on the ground. However, to properly comprehend how the sector functions an understanding of the landlord cohort, their motivations and behaviour, is essential.

This chapter therefore concentrates on the individuals and (in a few cases) companies who provide private rental housing in Australia, on the sector's evolving ownership structure, and on the market conditions and policy settings that have influenced this. Along the way we highlight many similarities, and some contrasts, with respect to private rental housing provision in Australia and in comparator countries.

A. Morris et al., *The Private Rental Sector in Australia*,
https://doi.org/10.1007/978-981-33-6672-5_3

The recent surge of private rental property investment in Australia and internationally can be linked with the broader global trend towards the financialisation of housing, as noted in Chap. 1. This refers to '… structural changes in housing and financial markets and global investment whereby housing is treated as a commodity, a means of accumulating wealth and often as security for financial instruments that are traded and sold on global markets' (Farha, 2017, p. 3). As implied by this comment, the past 20–30 years have seen dwellings coming to be viewed increasingly as tradeable assets rather than as homes.

Latterly, financialisation scholars have given increased attention to rental housing investment (Fields, 2014; DeWilde, 2018; Martin, 2018). Perhaps the most glaring instances of private rental financialisation concern the corporate investor acquisition of large property portfolios in certain European and North American cities, in some cases resulting in mass property upgrading and risks of population displacement (Fields & Uffer, 2016). While this latter phenomenon has yet to be seen in Australia, growing rental housing financialisation in our context is embodied in the changing 'calculative practices' and decision-making of individual small-scale landlords, as part of the financialisation of everyday life, as discussed later in this chapter.

The remainder of the chapter is structured as follows. In the next section we discuss the various forms of private landlordism—not just the distinction between companies, on the one hand, and individuals, on the other, but how the dominant mass of individual landlords may be usefully differentiated. Next, to help frame and explain the changing nature and scale of private rental housing investment we briefly review key influencing developments in global financial markets, as well as Australia's tax settings and regulatory levers that contribute towards shaping landlord behaviours. Having covered the market and policy context, we move to the chapter's centrepiece: an account of landlords' investment behaviour and motivations. The prime focus here is the nation's 2.1 million small-scale rental property owners who provide the vast bulk of Australia's mainstream PRS housing stock. However, recognising the possibility that it might come to form a significant sector component in future, institutionally-financed and owned 'build to rent' housing is also discussed. Then, in our penultimate section, we highlight the ways that emerging patterns of landlord activity are being reflected in changes to the spatial distribution of private rental housing in Australia's major cities; changes that are having increasingly significant impacts on our urban social geography. Finally, in conclusion we draw together key themes and implications from the main body of the chapter.

PRS Provision—Overview of Market Segments and Landlord Types

Private Rental Sub-Sectors

As intimated in Chaps. 1 and 2, Australia's PRS is properly understood as a diverse body of housing containing distinct sub-sectors located in different parts of the market and catering for different populations. Partly to provide a basis for the supply side analysis contained within this chapter, Table 3.1 identifies five broad sector components. In size, the 'mainstream' element is overwhelmingly dominant; to a greater or lesser extent, the other four elements are much smaller niche components. Accordingly, while most of this chapter is devoted to the mainstream part of the sector, we briefly comment below on each of these other sub-sectors.

Boarding houses, as referenced in Table 3.1, have historically tended to provide the most inexpensive (and basic) form of private rental accommodation. Here we are talking about the 'traditional' boarding (or, as in Victoria, rooming) house form containing multiple bedrooms provided on a furnished basis, with residents sharing communal facilities such as kitchens, bathrooms, laundries and living areas. Under state\territory-specific rules these are typically regulated within the terms of environmental health legislation, often with the involvement of local councils to oversee health and safety aspects. According to the latest Census, boarding house residents numbered some 17,500 across Australia in 2016 (ABS, 2018). In 2014 there were 1,905 registered boarding houses in NSW and Victoria, mainly located in Sydney and Melbourne (Dalton et al., 2015).

Distinct from traditional boarding (or rooming) houses as classified in Table 3.1 are the so-called New Generation Boarding Houses that have latterly burgeoned in Sydney under the NSW Government's 2009 Affordable Rental Housing State

Table 3.1 Australian private rental typology

Sub sector	Ownership	Market position	Tenant target group
Mainstream	Individual 'mum and dad' investors	Diverse	Diverse
Boarding houses	Individuals, companies	Low end	Low-income single people
Purpose-built student accommodation	Financial institutions, companies	Mid-market to high end	International and some domestic students
Mainstream build to rent	Financial Institutions, developers	High end	Young professionals, primarily non-families
Short stay rental	Individuals, including 'mum and dad investors'	Mid-market to high end	Tourists and mobile workers

Source Authors

Environment Planning Policy (ARHSEPP). Associated relaxation of certain standard planning expectations allowed construction of what are, in effect, rental micro-apartment blocks. Despite their official designation, these differ fundamentally from traditional boarding houses in that residents enjoy exclusive use of a private kitchen and bathroom. Physically, with unit floorspace typically around 25–30 square metres, such blocks have much in common with purpose-built student accommodation (PBSA) and are sometimes used as such. At the same time, the NGBH model can be seen as a precursor form of mainstream build to rent (BtR) housing. Both PBSA and mainstream BtR are more fully discussed later in this chapter.

A final PRS market component identified in Table 3.1 is the short-term letting sub-sector targeting tourists or temporary business visitors, and which has burst onto the scene during the past decade. Featuring a number of companies, of which AirBnB is only the most well-known, this involves the relatively unregulated renting out of residential rooms or entire apartments or houses for short-term occupancy. Such platforms have provided a flexible means for residential property owners to generate an income stream from their own home (by renting out a previously un-used room), or otherwise compounding existing income generation (by transitioning a mainstream rental property into the potentially more lucrative short-term letting market). At least for those happening to own real estate in desirable locations, this phenomenon can be argued as having contributed towards a new shift in favour of seeing residential property as an economic asset. As such it is widely considered a prime example of housing financialisation (Bernardi, 2018; Cocola-Gant & Gago, 2019).

By 2018, it was reported that AirBnB listings alone were running at over 20,000 in both Sydney and Melbourne (Crommelin et al., 2018). While viewed in a citywide context, these numbers are relatively small, their geographical concentration in city centre, beachside or similar areas makes them highly significant market components in such localities. Thus, especially to the extent that short-term letting involves whole dwellings rather than home-sharing (see Crommelin et al., 2018), they have sparked concerns around the resulting stress on already pressured rental housing markets (Parkinson et al., 2018; Wachsmuth et al., 2017). During 2020, the shutdown of international tourism due to the COVID-19 crisis placed in doubt the continued vitality of this sector. Substantial numbers of such homes filtered (back) into the mainstream market from which many originated. Whether this will represent an enduring re-set or a short-term crisis adjustment will of course depend partly on when, and to what extent, international tourism revives in the wake of the COVID-19 crisis.

Landlord Typologies

Different types of landlords will hold different types of property portfolios as well as pursuing varying investment and/or holding objectives. This diversity will likely influence the basis on which rental properties are offered for rent, in this way generating significant implications for the ways that PRS housing is experienced by tenants.

In differentiating private landlord entities, a traditional distinction has been made between employers,[1] companies and individuals. Beyond this, in relation to the individual small-scale investors who dominate rental housing provision in Australia and most comparator countries, efforts have been made to differentiate individual small-scale investors. As noted in Chap. 1, a basic distinction can be posed between 'accidental' and 'purposeful' landlords. The former are people renting out properties not originally acquired with this objective in mind. The most significant forms of accidental landlordism involve properties rented out by a former owner occupier, or upon inheritance. ABS surveys during the 1990s, the latest data available, suggested that *accidental landlords* accounted for around 30% of all individual landlords at that time (Beer, 1999; Berry, 2000). The numbers are likely to remain substantial today. Arguably, renting from an accidental landlord may place a tenant in a less secure position, since the property's rental use is more likely to be considered as a temporary measure (Wood & Ong, 2013; Rugg & Rhodes, 2018).

In contrast to accidental landlords, purposeful landlords involve people who can be more accurately be termed 'landlord investors' in the sense of having made a deliberate decision to acquire residential property (usually incurring mortgage debt, in the process) with the specific intention of renting it out.

Over and above the accidental versus purposeful distinction, there is no generally accepted classification of individual landlords. Some suggested taxonomies have highlighted the scale of investor operations. Following Allen and McDowell (1989), however, others have placed more emphasis on investor motivations, behaviour and characteristics. In part reflecting a UK historical perspective, Kemp (2015) distinguished between 'traditional' and 'buy to let' landlords—the former being 'cash-buyers' while the latter (nowadays ubiquitous) have financed their acquisition(s) largely or wholly through debt. Meanwhile, Rugg and Rhodes (2019) argue for a threefold classification of purposeful investors as 'pension plan landlords', 'portfolio-building landlords' or 'divesting landlords'. More simply, Soaita et al. (2017) differentiated the ambitious 'Property Ladder' strategists who prioritised leveraging of accumulating equity to expand portfolios, from the 'Why not? investors'—whose explanation for purchase of an investment property was simply 'everybody does it'.

---

[1] Employer-provided housing was a feature of some early industrial era societies in Europe and North America. It was also significant historically in Australia, in the form of public service employee housing provided by governments to facilitate regional office postings. Employer-provided housing remains present to this day in the very specific context of remote mining centres, albeit that its importance has been diminished by the fly-in-fly-out (FIFO) working regime.

Implicit in some of the above typologies is an attempt to distinguish between more professional versus more amateurish landlord motivations and behaviour which, once again, could have implications for tenant experiences. However, none of the research cited above has been conducted in Australia and Australian evidence on classification of individual landlords is very limited. Evidence on whether and how Australian private landlords might be classed within the amateur verse professional framework is discussed later in this chapter.

Australian Context for Rental Property Investment

In this section we first discuss the ways that global economic trends have arguably helped fuel the rise of housing financialisation, and the private rental housing investment boom that has been one of its effects. Building on Chap. 1, we then go on to explain the policy settings that also shape the business climate for investor landlord activity; in particular, the tax settings that famously provide such a favourable context for individual landlordism in Australia. Finally, the section briefly discusses the financial regulation levers recently deployed by Federal regulators in influencing investor landlord property acquisition activity.

Market Conditions

As noted in Chap. 1, a crucial starting point for Australia's private rental revival of the past 30 years was the deregulation of housing finance which freed up mortgage loans for rental housing acquisition from the mid-1980s. Especially from the mid-1990s, this has been compounded by a global dynamic of generally falling interest rates associated with the worldwide savings glut that began to be recognised at this time. As put by Belsky and Richardson (2010, p. 4), "a remarkable amount of cash began to look for opportunities for higher returns". This expanded the amount of mortgage finance available and reduced its cost (Kemp, 2015). At the same time, finance sector innovation and, from 2009, central bank pro-liquidity strategies, have also enabled the expansion of credit-fuelled landlord expenditure on rental property.

The growing investment attractiveness of housing, especially over the past 10–20 years, reflects the post-millennial decline of financial yields typically recorded in other investment asset classes—most particularly commercial property and the share market (Pawson & Milligan, 2013; Pawson et al., 2019). It is not that rental housing returns (the ratio of rents to property values) have significantly improved. Rather, gradually falling returns from competing asset classes have been diminishing the yield gap between such asset classes and housing—historically a large gulf, but latterly an increasingly narrow margin. This has stimulated interest among institutional investors (e.g. superannuation funds and insurance companies in residential rental—build to rent housing—as a possible new investment vehicle). However, for reasons explained later in this chapter, institutional investment currently continues to account for only a small proportion of PRS investment in Australia.

Similarly, the fund managers who influence investment capital deployment decisions have become more sensitised to the benefits of holding a low risk (even if relatively low yield) component within broader asset portfolios (Pawson & Milligan, 2013). In part this reflects the experience of growing share market volatility over the past 10–20 years, not only during worldwide crises such as the GFC and the COVID-19 economic crash. This accords with evidence on individual landlords in Australia and elsewhere (Isaac, 1998; Berry, 2000; Seelig et al., 2009; others) which points to a belief in the solidity of 'bricks and mortar' over other types of financial investments which can carry higher risk.

Tax Settings

Having sketched the economic backdrop to landlord investor activity over recent decades, we now move on to outline the key policy settings that frame landlord property acquisition and holding decisions in Australia. As mentioned in Chap. 1, the most important of these are the federal government tax rules concerning Capital Gains Tax and so-called negative gearing. These concessions, in combination, direct an effective subsidy to landlords through the reduction of investors' income tax liability—at an annual cost (tax revenue foregone) estimated at between $7.7 billion and $11.7 billion (Grudnoff, 2015; Daley et al., 2016). Especially since (as shown in Fig. 3.5) most private rental property investment involves acquisition of existing (not newly-built) dwellings, this is inflationary—being applied to a product subject to inelastic supply, subsidies are capitalised into higher house prices.[2]

As outlined in Chap. 1, negative gearing is the practice whereby landlords may write off expenses related to their investment property (e.g. mortgage interest payments and other holding costs), against their *entire income*, including income from unrelated activities such as an employee salary.[3] It enables an otherwise-employed landlord incurring a net loss on their rental property (outgoings exceeding rental income) to reduce the tax otherwise payable on their salary (or profits if a business owner). Where it operates in this way, such a device is sometimes termed a tax shelter. Negative gearing is therefore especially beneficial for higher tax-rate payers.

---

[2]This refers to the way that expectations on 'profitability' (or net return on investment) are factored into the market value of assets such as rental housing. For example, even before its implementation, a property tax change announcement will likely affect the prices that purchasers will be willing to pay for asset acquisitions.

[3]Importantly, it must be stressed that the facility to deduct business expenses from associated taxable income is a standard tax system principle designed to encourage investment (it is not restricted to rental housing). However, as argued by the Grattan Institute 'there is no in-principle reason why losses on investments should be deductible from entirely unrelated income such as wages' (Daley et al., 2016, p. 22).

Far from being a recent tax provision, or one specific to rental housing, Australian tax rules enabling negative gearing in this context have existed since the 1920s. However, the Hawke government's (ultimately reversed) 1985 efforts to remove the tax sheltering provisions of negative gearing substantially raised its profile as a financially attractive landlord business practice (Burke, 2012; Hulse & Burke, 2015). 'Subsequently, and in the context of broader financial deregulation, an industry of brokers, marketers and property advisors emerged using negative gearing as the hook to attract investors into the residential property sector' (Hulse et al., 2012, p. 18).

Capital Gains Tax (CGT) was introduced in Australia in 1985 to recover part of the unearned income derived from appreciating assets, or as explained by Beer (1999, p. 260), 'to stop wealthy individuals avoiding taxation by diverting income into capital-generating schemes'. Although initially charged at a taxpayer's marginal rate of income tax, a 50% CGT discount on the profit gleaned from the sale of an investment property was introduced in 1999. Fuller discussion of the rationale for this change, as well as the wider arguments for and against reform of landlord tax concessions can be found elsewhere (e.g. in Blunden 2016; Daley et al., 2016; Pawson et al., 2020).

Narratives Around Rental Property Ownership

Central in campaigns to resist calls for scaling back landlord tax concessions have been property industry efforts to shape popular narratives around rental property ownership. Hulse et al. (2019, p. 16) trace this back to the 1980s when the reframing of landlords as rental investors was boosted by the 1985–1987 debate on the reform of negative gearing. Since that time 'investor-landlordism has been valorized politically and normalized culturally as 'mum and dad rental investment' with connotations of enterprise and self-sufficiency rather than landlordism which has a more negative image'. Thus, landlords have been 'framed as Everyman, the archetypal person trying to get ahead in life' (Hulse et al., 2019, p. 7). Akin to John Howard's[4] noble 'battlers' this has a huge resonance in a society that traditionally venerates individualism and untrammelled property rights (Pawson, 2019). The limited extent to which the Everyman portrayal squares with statistical evidence on landlords' economic status is explored later in this chapter.

Illustrating the way that entitlement to tax-privileged wealth accumulation via rental property investment is understood by many as an inviolable and socially beneficial right, an audience member in ABC TV's Q&A program[5] in 2019 posed the following question to the panel:

[4]John Howard was the Prime Minister of Australia from 1996 to 2007. He led a right of centre Coalition government.

[5]Q and A is screened by the Australian Broadcasting Corporation (ABC). The format involves a moderator and a panel of experts and politicians who take questions from a studio audience.

> I bought my first property – negatively geared – when I was 17. By the time I was 23 I had two, which helped me buy my first family home. Thankfully, I hope that when I retire, I'll be off the social system. I'm also now trying to help my 17 year old son buy his first property so that hopefully one day he can also be off the social system…[W]hy would we take away something that … has been a great vehicle for many people to get into the investment market – to get into the property market? That [owner occupation] [is] one of things a Labor Government is actually talking about wanting the young to be able to get into … why would you take this vehicle away? (ABC Q&A, 29 April 2019)

The context for the question was the tax reform pledge adopted by the opposition Australian Labor Party in its (losing) platform for the 2016 Federal election, and as retained for the 2019 poll. This proposed the future restriction of negative gearing to newly-built housing. Similarly, the prevailing CGT discount would be halved for all newly-purchased rental properties. All existing rental property ownership would be grandfathered (i.e. rendered exempt from the reform). However, the proposals came under heavy fire in the lead-up to the ALP's losing 2019 election campaign, mainly on the grounds that any paring back of existing subsidies would risk 'a housing market crash' (Clench & Farr, 2018).

Before concluding this review of official policy settings that provide the context for rental property investment in Australia, we should briefly mention state/territory land taxes. As levied by all Australia's states, and the ACT, land tax is an annual charge set according to the value of land a taxpayer owns within the jurisdiction, subject to significant exemptions—most importantly, for owner occupiers. Crucially, the minimum land value thresholds below which owners are exempt, mean that the vast majority of individual landlords (because of owning only a single rental property) are zero-rated. As a result, such liability falls mainly on commercial property, and some rental housing (e.g. dwellings in the ownership of landlords with multiple properties).

The land tax structures described above are likely to have perpetuated what Berry (2000, p. 663) termed Australia's tradition of 'petty landlordism'. As he explained, 'In larger metropolitan markets the [rental property ownership] threshold is normally surpassed after one or, at most, two dwellings, encouraging the maintenance of a highly dispersed pattern of rental ownership'. This dynamic has recently come to the fore, in the context of developer-promoted build to rent projects that are disadvantaged as a result—as discussed below.

Financial Regulation and the PRS

Reference has already been made to the critical stimulus for rental sector revival provided by new regulatory settings for housing finance put in place in the 1980s. At present the responsible federal entity in such matters is the Australian Prudential Regulation Authority (APRA). Recent years have seen APRA wielding its powers over lending institutions to address concerns about investor landlord-driven house price booms (Pawson et al., 2020, p. 190). In 2014 and again in 2017, APRA imposed temporary restrictions on lenders specifically targeted on issuance of interest-only loans—the favoured form of mortgage for investor landlords. Both interventions registered significant market-cooling impacts, demonstrating the efficacy of financial regulation in this sphere (Morris, 2019).

Australia's Private Landlords: Property Portfolios and Investment Behaviour

Private Rental Property Ownership

In common with most comparator countries, private rental housing in Australia is overwhelmingly in the hands of individuals or couples with small property portfolios. As shown in Fig. 3.1, 58% of PRS properties are owned by Australia-resident landlords holding one or two rental dwellings only. Looked at in relation to households owning rental dwellings (rather than the ownership of the rental housing stock), very small-scale ownership appears to be even more dominant, since 70% of all households with rental properties owned just one such dwelling—see Fig. 3.2. Notably, this proportion has declined only slightly since the 1990s: as enumerated by ABS 1993 landlord survey, for example, 78% of individual rental property owners held a single property only (Beer, 1999).

Unfortunately, owing to imperfect data, there is uncertainty about the exact ownership status of the one fifth of all private rental dwellings labelled in Fig. 3.1 as relating to 'other owners'. These will include those owned by households with more four rental units and those held by overseas-based individuals, as well as those under

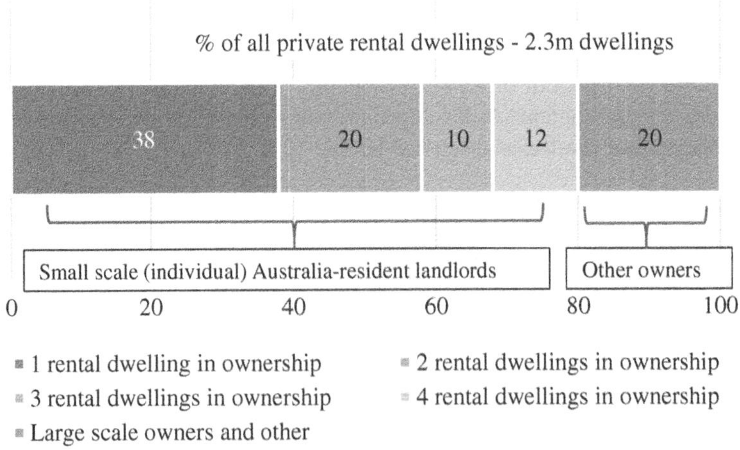

Fig. 3.1 Private rental dwellings in Australia by ownership in 2015–2016 (*Source* Pawson et al. [2020]; drawing on Hulse et al. [2019], Figure 2 which used customised data from ABS Survey of Income and Housing 2015–2016)

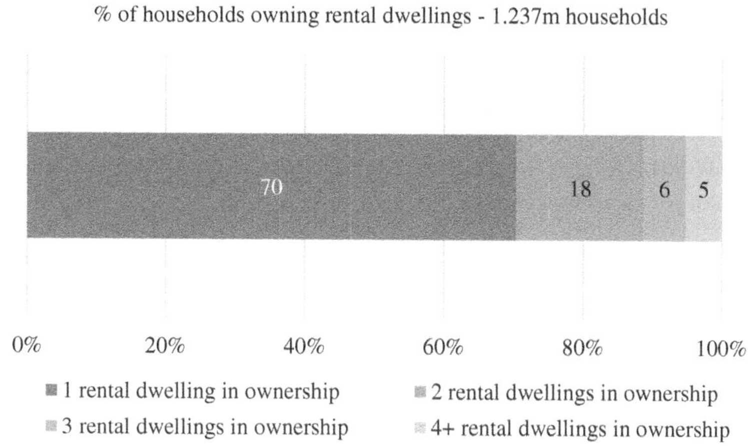

Fig. 3.2 Australia-resident households owning rental properties: breakdown by number owned (*Source* Draws on Hulse et al. [2019], Figure 2 using data from ABS Survey of Income and Housing 2015–2016)

other forms of private landlord entity—e.g. property companies, employers or trusts. The latter will include some held by self-managed super funds (SMSFs), a tax-advantaged investment vehicle set up to benefit an individual taxpayer or family. If SMSF holding is treated as a form of household (rather than corporate) ownership, and bearing in mind the likely significance of Australian individual landlords living overseas, the proportion of all private rental dwellings held by individuals may be much higher than 80%.

Landlord Incomes

In the remainder of this section we first explore in greater depth the profile of Australia's (non-corporate) private rental property owners.[6] Drawing on a range of evidence, Hulse et al. (2018, p. 4) usefully epitomise Australia's rental investors in the statement that a typical landlord is 'an owner occupier, at mid-life, in a household with two incomes'. The relatively high-income norm for this group is indicated by Table 3.2, demonstrating that both at the tax-payer (individual) level and the household level, landlords are a relatively advantaged group overall.

In support of the Everyman trope as earlier discussed, advocates of existing landlord tax concessions have often advanced dubious claims that, because investment property ownership is nowadays (allegedly) an ordinary person's pursuit, any change to current rules would inequitably 'hit working people'. Where backed by any

[6] Unfortunately, there has been no twenty-first century repeat of ABS landlord surveys undertaken in the 1990s (in 1993 and 1997). As a result, the main (albeit limited) sources for this section are Australian Tax Office records and the ABS Survey of Income and Housing.

Table 3.2 Individual rental property owners: income metrics

		Rental property owners	Others
Individual taxpayers (ATO)	*N*	2,108,550	11,373,400
Mean annual taxable income ($)		81,034	54,356
Households (SIH)	*N*	1,236,276	7,726,025
Mean annual gross household income ($)		175,387	98,799
Mean annual disposable household income ($)		135,392	81,598

Source Hulse et al. (2019), Table 1 using ATO 2% sample unit record file of individual tax returns, 2015–2016; and ABS Survey of Income and Housing, 2015–2016

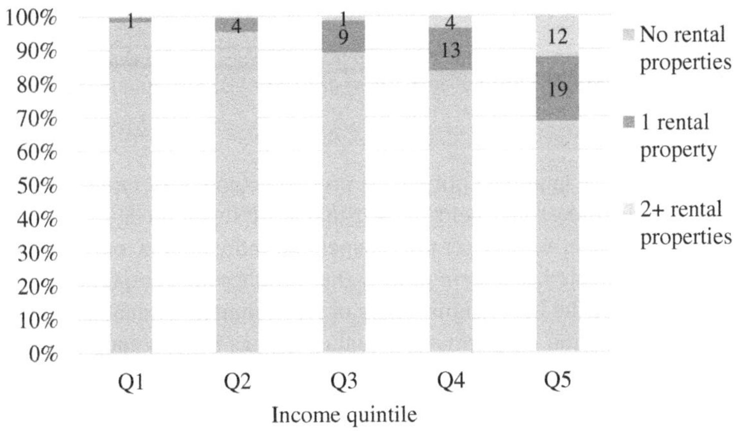

Fig. 3.3 Rental property-owning households by income quintile, 2013–2014 (*Source* Derived from Hulse et al. [2018], Table 3 based on data from ABS Survey of Income and Housing 2013–2014. *Note* Refers to household incomes after negative gearing has been applied)

supporting evidence, such claims have tended to rest on citation of taxable income statistics. On this basis it can be suggested that Australia in fact sees significant levels of rental property ownership among middle income households. However, this is something of a self-fulfilling prophecy, since the negative gearing rules themselves have the effect of disproportionately depressing investors' taxable incomes.

For the reasons explained above, it is gross (pre-tax) incomes—as analysed in Table 3.2—that provide a more meaningful foundation for assessing landlords' income profile. Further, as illustrated by Fig. 3.3, while rental property ownership is modestly represented among middle income earners, landlordism is far more common among more affluent groups. More starkly, while almost one in three top quintile income households hold at least one rental property, this is true for only one in a hundred lowest quintile earners.

These realities are confirmed by the Household Income and Labour Dynamics in Australia (HILDA) survey which illustrate that Quintile 1 and 2 income earners accounted for 13% of rental property owners in 2014, while Quintile 4 and 5 members made up 79%. Interestingly, the HILDA data for the period 2006–2014 also provide no evidence for any suggestion that rental property ownership is extending further down the income spectrum over time. The proportion of investor landlords classed as Q1/Q2 income earners remained more-or-less static over this period (Wilkins, 2016).

Given all of this evidence it is hardly surprising that investor landlord tax concessions disproportionately benefit higher income earners and the wealthy. Thus, some 50% of negative gearing concessions flow to the top 20% of households ranked by income (Grudnoff, 2018). Moreover, as estimated by the Grattan Institute, 80% of the value of CGT discount flows to the top 10% of income earners (Mather, 2018).

Corporate Landlords and Build to Rent

Although they remain niche players in Australia, the significance of corporate landlords has increased over the past 10–20 years. Here we are talking about rental housing funded and owned by financial institutions such as superannuation (or pension) funds, insurance companies and sovereign wealth funds. 'Build to rent' (BtR) is the term which has recently come into use in Australia (imported from the UK) to describe purpose-built apartment blocks to be held, long-term, in single ownership as rental housing. Such a move would indicate a shift from a develop/build and sell model to a develop/build and retain model for apartment blocks as represented in many other parts of the world.

As noted earlier in this chapter, the prospect that a mainstream BtR sector might emerge in Australia appears to have been brought somewhat closer by the relative improvement in rental housing financial rates of return seen over the past two decades. Since around 2017, this prospect has generated intense development industry interest and lobbying activity—partly inspired by a growing appreciation that a flourishing BtR construction sector has functioned for decades in North America (where it is known as 'multi-family housing'), and that BtR has more recently made a strong emergence in the UK (Pawson et al., 2019).

Arguably, BtR offers potential to fulfil certain significant public policy objectives. From the consumer perspective, the possible emergence of purpose-built, professionally-managed rental housing could raise management and maintenance standards and broaden choice. Moreover, tenants may benefit from a greater sense of security than the current rental market norm, where—in a market dominated by individual landlord investors primarily motivated by capital gains—there is an ever-present possibility of tenancy termination to facilitate property sale (Wood & Ong, 2013).

At the same time, at least in its initial Australian incarnation, mainstream (i.e. non-student) BtR provision will not cater for low to moderate income renters. Rather, it has been generally interpreted by developers in the field as a fairly high-end product that will involve large schemes sited in relatively prestigious locations and primarily targeted at young professionals (Pawson et al., 2019). This is related to the 'premium market' status of early adopter BtR development industry players and lobbyists. It also follows from the inspiration of US multi-family housing projects which tend to cater for an up-market tenant population.

Over time, the tenant target group might reach a little further down the income spectrum—some developers interviewed in our 2019 research believed that having established 'proof of concept' through an initial upmarket offer, future BtR projects could become more diverse in terms of market targeting and location. However, under prevailing Australian housing market conditions and policy settings, and in the absence of government subsidy, there was little or no scope for building rental housing affordable to lower income tenants through market BtR schemes. Moreover, as demonstrated by development feasibility modelling, governments seeking to facilitate such provision (and willing to pledge the necessary subsidy) would be well-advised to utilise not-for-profit community housing providers (rather than for-profit developers) for this purpose (Pawson et al., 2019).

Since 2018 a scattering of Australian mainstream BtR projects have been announced by a few large developers. However, partly reflecting various tax system disadvantages (see land tax discussion above), the financial feasibility of such a product currently remains highly marginal, and in the absence of significant changes in market conditions and/or tax settings[7] it seems unlikely that BtR will take off in any major way (Pawson et al., 2019).

Nevertheless, a BtR variant—purpose-built student housing (PBSA)—has already acquired a major presence in Australia. Essentially, PBSA is institutionally-financed accommodation held in single ownership as tenanted housing for long-term rental revenue generation. As in many other countries the sector has expanded rapidly in Australia since the 1990s, in this case aided by government support in the form of guaranteed income agreements as well as tax and planning concessions and a high demand from international students who numbered 565,000 by 2020 (Australian Government, 2020). By 2019, PBSA bedspaces in Australia totalled some 86,000, projected to exceed 100,000 by 2022 (JLL, 2019). Much of this development has been underwritten by overseas-based pension funds and sovereign wealth entities; the kinds of players who could come to emerge as significant stakeholders in the mainstream rental market if BtR were to take off in a broader sense. At the time of writing, there are questions about whether the short-term decline in student enrolment

[7] A potentially important 2020 development in this arena has been the NSW Government's announcement of a land tax concession for owners of large BtR schemes. Under the proposal (Scheule, 2020), qualifying BtR landlords will be entitled to a 50% discount on land tax otherwise payable. This is likely to significantly enhance the financial feasibility of mainstream BtR projects in Australia's largest state, although without other "playing field levelling" changes in national tax settings (see Pawson et al., 2019), it is unlikely to prove decisive.

due to the COVID-19 crisis proves a precursor to a more sustained downturn in the number of international students.

Investor Landlord Motivations and Behaviour

For the past 30 years, private rental investors have formed a large body of Australia's house purchase demand. As conventionally measured—in terms of the proportion of total mortgage finance being issued—investor landlords accounted for 37% of property purchasers over the period 2003–2019 (ABS, 2020).

As indicated in Fig. 3.4, the period 2011–2017 saw a major spike in investor property acquisition activity. The first three years of this period saw a 68% increase in mortgage loans issued to investors, a surge in rental property homebuying that hugely contributed to the house price boom seen at this time (Lane, 2019). This was especially so in Australia's two largest cities—Sydney and Melbourne. On an annual basis, investor finance peaked in 2014 at 43% of total housing loans issued during the year. Especially from 2017, investor lending fell back sharply, partly as a result of regulatory intervention by APRA as discussed earlier in this chapter (Pawson et al., 2020).

By comparison with home owners, rental investors form a potentially more volatile component of housing market demand. Logic would suggest that this is true not only in relation to their property acquisition behaviour, but also their portfolio-holding decisions. For an investor landlord, decisions on when to buy and sell are not influenced by the sentimental attachment felt to one's own home nor by experiences

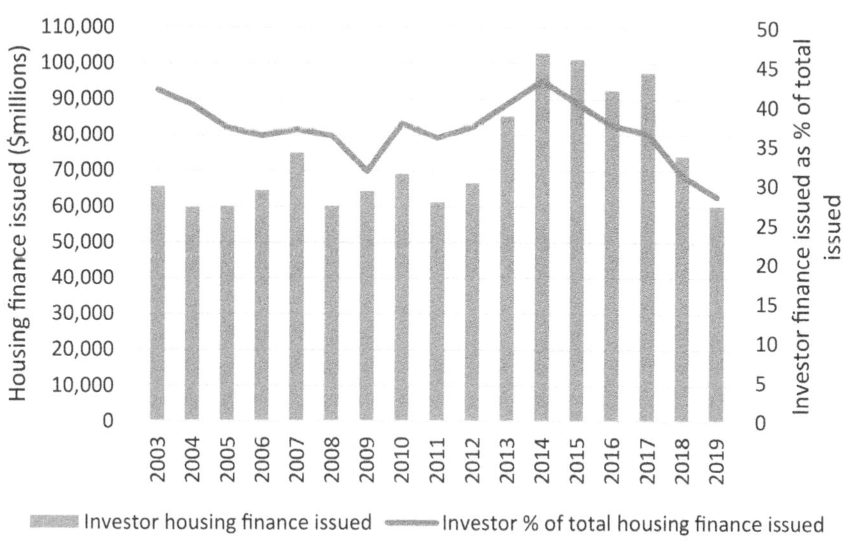

Fig. 3.4 Housing loan finance issued to rental investors, 2002–2019 (*Source* ABS Lending Indicators, Cat 5601: Tables 4 and 14)

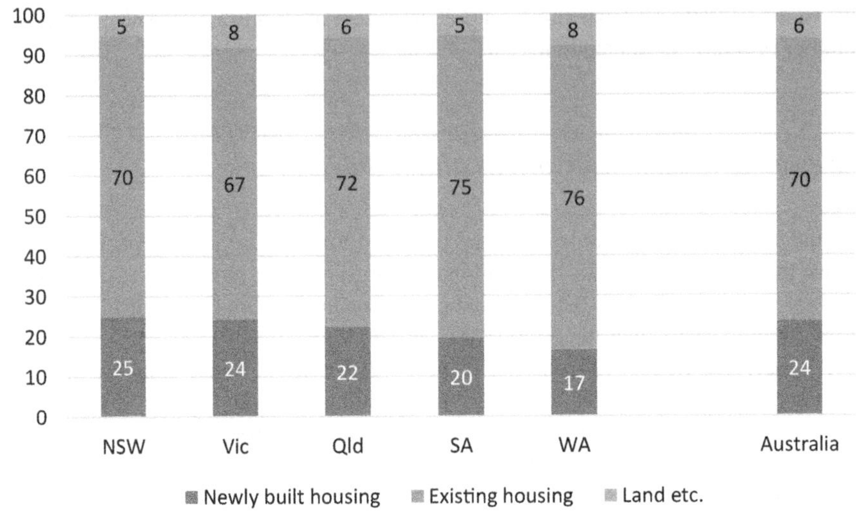

Fig. 3.5 Investor landlord loan finance issued Jul 2019–Jan 2020: property type breakdown (*Source* ABS Lending Indicators, Cat 5601: Tables 15–19)

of living there. Even under the strengthened provisions for tenant security recently enacted by the Victorian Government (see Chap. 2), there is no impediment to a landlord wanting to end a tenancy and marketing their property for sale with vacant possession. With these considerations in mind, therefore, many have expressed concern that a serious market downturn could prompt large scale rental property sell-offs, with disruptive resulting effects for tenants.

While these anxieties cannot be entirely dismissed, available research evidence suggests that small-scale landlord rental housing acquisitions are generally predicated on an assumption of long-term property holding (Seelig et al., 2009). In the last major national study of landlords undertaken in Australia, Seelig and colleagues concluded that age and personal circumstances—rather than market conditions—were the dominant factors influencing the likelihood of future property sale. Complementing this finding, panel survey evidence indicates that the propensity to dispose of rental property is strongly related to landlord age: '…once retired there is a sharp increase in the likelihood of exit from rental investments' (Wood & Ong, 2013, p. 3243).

Although published evidence is thin, it would appear that at least until fairly recently, investor landlord behaviour on rental property acquisition has generally remained largely amateur and risk averse rather than professional and entrepreneurial. Thus, as reported by Seelig and colleagues referencing rental investors of the 2000s: 'sentimentality and informality appear to be important… Personal experience and intuition are reported as the dominant sources of information for investors in making property investment decisions' (Seelig et al., 2009, p. 2). Similar findings were reached by UK research evidence of that pre-electronic-property-market era (Crook et al., 2009).

In Australia, over the last decade, however, the growth in private rental investment has been accompanied by a burgeoning industry of "property investment advisors, residential investment magazines and home investment and renovation television shows" (Hulse et al., 2012, p. 22). This has been underpinned by an electronic property data revolution, enabling online sales price histories, virtual property tours, investment blogs and seminars (Martin, 2018). It would be expected that such infrastructure could well have made a marked impact on Australia's small landlord culture both in promoting the idea of being a "property investor" rather than a landlord (Hulse et al., 2019) and in shaping property purchase decisions. This could mean investors engaging in what has been termed "borderless investment"—buying in regional centres or outside of their home states based on the availability of digital property information (Hulse et al., 2018, p. 30).

More recent evidence on landlord behaviour does suggest that in the past 10–15 years there may have been a significant shift towards a more "business savvy" approach to private landlordism in this country. A study of rental investors in western Sydney (Western Sydney property investor, cited in Pawson & Martin, 2020), found indications of a distinctly more financialised mindset than that described by Seelig et al. (2009) and other earlier researchers. Growing an investment property portfolio for capital gain was the predominant motivation across our landlord cohort although investors were also attentive to rental returns. With little expressed intention to trade or flip properties short-term, many landlords were following a business strategy of using capital growth to lever into further property acquisitions. This would imply investors more aggressively using debt and more actively growing and managing property portfolios than the 'mum and dad landlords' of yesteryear. Some of these points are illustrated by the following quotes from rental investors in western Sydney, as interviewed in 2017 in connection with a research project cited above (Hulse et al., 2019; Pawson & Martin, 2020)[8]:

> [I] buy something that I can add value to through adding a granny flat, and refinancing...the trick is that once you do that, you add one fifty thousand onto that property, you want to be able to build that back out. So after you've done renovation the property has increased in value, then you go with a valuation on it and refinance and draw out that money you put in it, and then move on to the next property. As long as the banks continue lending to you. (Western Sydney rental property investor, 2017)

> I invested in many ... states, to reduce land tax , and also to spread risk... I use equity in properties I already own, extending debt to buy more [by leveraging] existing properties to get 20% deposit or sometimes less and then pay Lenders Mortgage Insurance. (Western Sydney rental property investor, 2017)

> I read a lot of books ... about what to look for in an investment area, demographics, infrastructure ... enough research to make emotionally detached decisions. (Western Sydney rental property investor, 2017)

Important in terms of the housing market impacts of rental investor activity is the property acquisition choices landlords make on property types and locations. As indicated in Fig. 3.5, acquired properties are predominantly existing—rather than newly-built—homes. Moreover, the differences from state to state are fairly modest.

[8]Quotes 2 and 3 are cited from the Pawson and Martin (2020) paper.

Unfortunately, because the relevant data series commenced only during 2019, it is not yet possible to track any changes over time on this measure.

The Changing Geography of Australia's Private Rental Housing

Historically, as in many comparator countries, private rental populations in Sydney, Melbourne and other major cities were strongly concentrated in inner urban locations as discussed in Chap. 1. Over the past 30 years, however, private landlords' property acquisition and property holding behaviour have resulted in a distinct outward shift. The anatomy of this change for Sydney and Melbourne is indicated in Fig. 3.6.

The relative suburbanisation of private rental housing seen in cities like Sydney and Melbourne since the 1980s will have been partly driven by the 'gentrification' of many inner suburbs, where formerly rented properties have been renovated or replaced in the course of a transition to owner occupation (Bounds & Morris, 2006). At the same time, it appears that private rental investors have increasingly looked to the middle and outer suburbs as attractive sites for property acquisition.[9]

A key factor likely underlying the urban restructuring implied by Fig. 3.6 is the relatively high rental yields (ratio of rental income to property value) typical for many middle and outer suburban locations. This, in turn, reflects the fact that city-wide variation in rent levels is less than differentials on sale prices—that is, the centre-to-periphery gradient for rental prices is flatter than for purchase prices (Hulse et al., 2014). Renting in an outer suburb of Sydney or Melbourne is usually cheaper than in the inner city, but the difference is not as great as the inner/outer suburb difference in property values. Relatively high rates of private rental property growth in middle and outer suburbs also reflects contemporary market conditions and investor landlord behaviour. In our sample of property acquiring rental investors in western Sydney, only one in seven lived locally, while almost one in five lived at least 40 km distant.

In many cases remote landlordism of this kind is facilitated by landlords' use of real estate agents to manage their properties and their relationships with private renters. About seven in ten privately rented properties in Australia are managed by real estate agents (Martin et al., p. 47) such that most landlords are hands-off in terms of management of their properties and addressing renter concerns. The responsiveness of agents to tenants' concerns has become a key issue in thinking about the future of private renting as we discuss in the last chapter of this book. In relying on intermediaries in this way, the Australian PRS differs from some other countries,

[9]Much of this will have involved dwellings built, and previously used as, owner occupied homes. For example, our previously mentioned western Sydney study found that this was true of 38% of properties acquired for rental use in the period 2011–2015 (Pawson & Martin, 2020, Table 6).

(a) Sydney

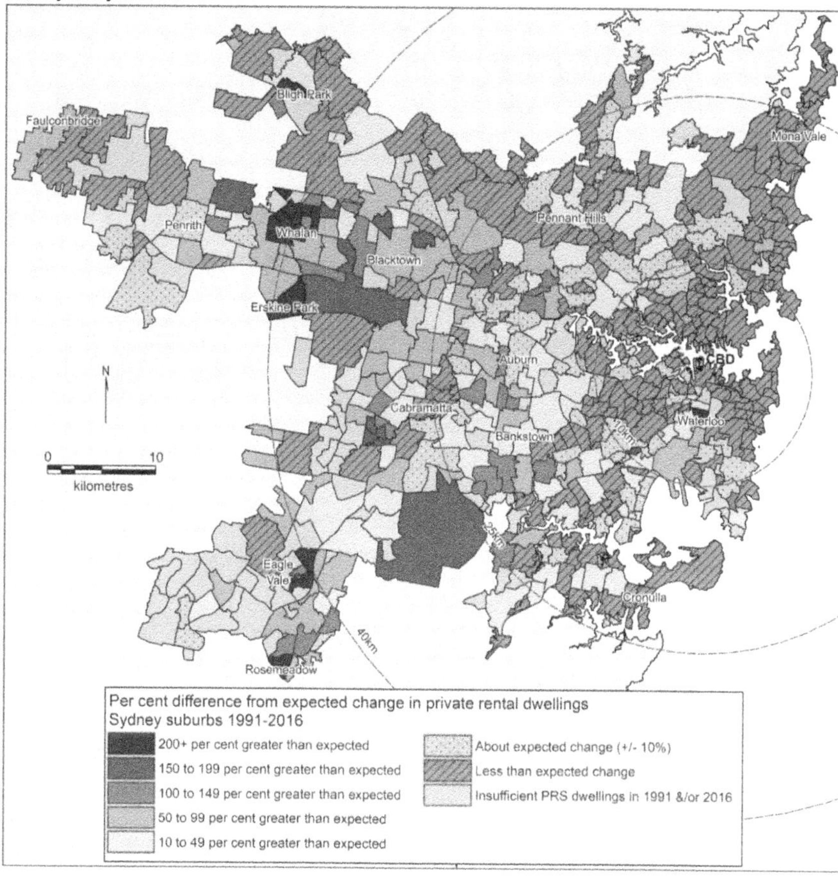

Fig. 3.6 Shift-share analysis: difference between expected and actual change in private rental populations, 1991–2016 (*Source* ABS 1991 and 2016 Census. Map credit: Margaret Reynolds, Swinburne University of Technology. *Notes* Maps (a) and (b) show the shift-share of private rental in each metropolitan Sydney and Melbourne suburb (synonymous with 'neighbourhood' in this context) from 1991 to 2016. That is, it shows the extent to which the growth in private rental as a tenure share compares with an 'expected' growth in private rental over that period. Expectation is set by both the tenure share in each suburb at the beginning of the period and the metropolitan-wide change in tenure share over the period. For a fuller explanation of shift-share analysis see Loveridge and Selting [1998])

particularly in Europe, where management by the landlord is more common (Martin et al., 2018).

(b) Melbourne

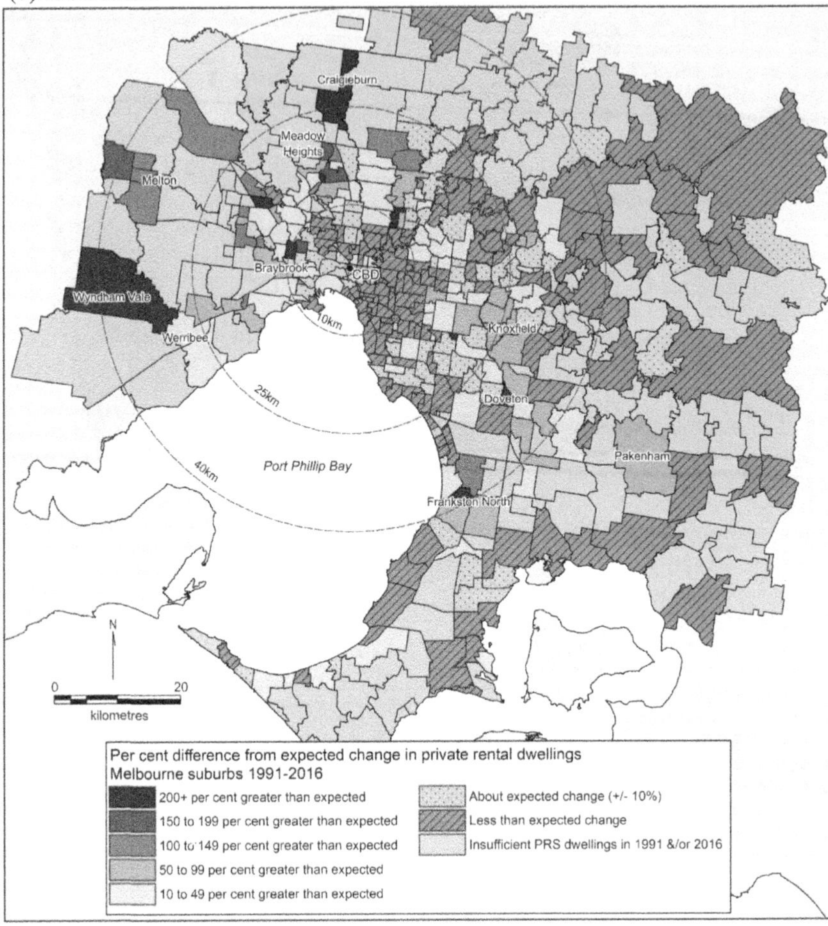

Fig. 3.6 (continued)

More detailed analysis of long-term spatial shifts in private rental metropolitan provision shows that the pattern of change also reflects local socio-economic status. Thus, the most grossly disproportionate expansion in private rental housing recorded in Sydney over the 25 years to 2016 was in areas that were *both* distant from the CBD (30 km or more) and ranked in the most socio-economically disadvantaged cohort of suburbs in 1991. Connecting the changing urban geography of disadvantage with the behaviour of landlord investors, Hulse and Reynolds (2018) coined the term 'investification' to capture this connection wherein patterns of private rental investment contribute to changes in the distribution of socio-economic disadvantage.

All of this needs to be seen within the context of the already well-documented tendency for the outward shift of low income populations in Australia's major cities, a tendency termed 'the suburbanisation of disadvantage' (Randolph & Holloway, 2005; Randolph & Tice, 2016). The housing market is funnelling the low-income tenants who depend on private rental housing away from inner urban locations and into areas more remote from the inner city epicentres of high value employment growth.

Noteworthy is that the niche private rental sub-sectors identified in Table 3.1 all have their own specific geographies. The boarding house sector, disproportionately represented in big cities, is largely an inner-city phenomenon in Sydney, whereas in Melbourne it is concentrated in South Eastern suburbs. Mainstream BtR housing, as it has begun to emerge in Australia, tends to be associated with inner urban sites close to good transport links. Short stay rental housing (e.g. AirBnB) has been strongly concentrated in beachside or inner urban locations (Crommelin et al., 2018). Although their numbers remain relatively small if viewed at the metropolitan scale, this geography means that in certain suburbs their numbers are very substantial—with the potential to make a significant impact on local rental housing markets, compounding pressures on any lower income renters remaining in such areas.

Conclusions

The story of Australia's private landlords and rental housing stock is largely one relating to household investment in established dwellings physically indistinguishable from owner occupied properties. It is a story that has seen a progressively more financialised landlord mindset where investment choices appear increasingly informed by unsentimental decision-making which focuses more single-mindedly on rental return and capital value uplift. While not quite the uniquely landlord-friendly tax environment that is sometimes portrayed, Australia's relatively generous tax treatment of landlords has continued to support this culture. Casting this in particularly sharp relief is the relatively light regulatory protection enjoyed by tenants.

With the niche exception of purpose-built student housing, individuals (rather than companies) continue to dominate Australia's private rental ownership structure. Recent decades of sector growth have also seen the ongoing predominance of single-property-owning landlords. Multi-property landlordism has also been expanding but only at a similar rate. Whether a mainstream market version of build to rent development will become established in the 2020s is not yet certain.

Uncertainties of far larger magnitude relate to the duration of the COVID-19 triggered halt to international tourism and migration—each of which have formed crucial drivers of private rental growth in recent years. During 2020, a resulting glut of supply and dearth of demand in many inner-city and beachside suburbs of Melbourne and Sydney saw market conditions decisively favouring tenants over landlords—a situation rarely witnessed in modern urban Australia.

References

ABC TV. (2019). *Q&A 29 April*. https://www.abc.net.au/qanda/2019-29-04/11037644.

ABS (Australian Bureau of Statistics). (2018). *Census of population and housing: Estimating homelessness, 2016*. Cat 2049.0, https://www.abs.gov.au/AUSSTATS/abs@.nsf/allprimarymainfeatures/ED457E1CF56EA15ECA257A7500148DB3?opendocument.

ABS (Australian Bureau of Statistics). (2020). *Lending indicators*. Cat 5601.0, https://www.abs.gov.au/ausstats/abs@.nsf/mf/5601.0.

Australian Government (2020). *Coronavirus and temporary visa holders*. https://minister.homeaffairs.gov.au/davidcoleman/Pages/Coronavirus-and-Temporary-Visa-holders.aspx.

Beer, A. (1999). Housing investment in the private rental sector in Australia. *Urban Studies, 36*(2), 255–269.

Belsky, E., & Richardson, N. (2010). *Understanding the boom and bust in nonprime mortgage lending*. Cambridge, MA: Joint Centre for Housing Studies of Harvard University.

Bernardi, M. (2018). The impact of AirBnB on our cities: Gentrification and 'disneyfication' 2.0, *Urban Media Lab*, 2 October, https://labgov.city/theurbanmedialab/the-impact-of-airbnb-on-our-cities-gentrification-and-disneyfication-2-0/.

Berry, M. (2000). Investment in rental housing in Australia: Small landlord and institutional investors. *Housing Studies, 15*(5), 661–681.

Blunden, H. (2016). Discourses around negative gearing of investment properties in Australia. *Housing Studies, 31*(3), 340–357.

Bounds, M., & Morris, A. (2006). Second wave gentrification in inner-city Sydney. *Cities, 23*(2), 99–108.

Burke, T. (2012). The Australian residential housing market: Institutions and actors. In R. Tomlinson (Ed.), *Australia's unintended cities*. Melbourne: CSIRO.

Clench, S., & Farr, M. (2018, September 19). 'Inviting a crash': PM issues ominous warning as he defends government's housing policies, *News.com.au*. https://tinyurl.com/y5tpcrlq.

Cocola-Gant, A., & Gago, A. (2019). Airbnb, buy-to-let investment and tourism-driven displacement: A case study in Lisbon. *Environment and Planning: Economy and Space*. https://doi.org/10.1177/0308518X19869012.

Crook, A. D. H., Kemp, P. A., & Ferrari, E. (2009). *Views and experiences of landlords in the private rented sector*. Edinburgh: Scottish Government.

Crommelin, L., Troy, L., Martin, C., & Parkinson, S. (2018). *Technological disruption in private housing markets: The case of Airbnb* (Final Report 305). Melbourne: AHURI.

Daley, J., Wood, D., & Parsonage, H. (2016). *Hot property negative gearing and capital gains tax reform*. Melbourne: Grattan Institute.

Dalton, T., Pawson, H., & Hulse, K. (2015). *Rooming house futures: Governing for growth, fairness and transparency*, No 245. Melbourne: Australian Housing and Urban Research Institute (AHURI).

Dewilde, C. (2018). Explaining the declined affordability of housing for low-income private renters across Western Europe. *Urban Studies, 55*(12), 2618–2639. https://doi.org/10.1177/0042098017729077.

Farha, L. (2017). *Report of the Special Rapporteur on adequate housing*. United Nations General Assembly, Human Rights Council, 34th Session 27 February–24 March. https://documents.un.org/prod/ods.nsf/xpSearchResultsM.xsp.

Fields, D. (2014). *The rise of the corporate landlord: The institutionalisation of the single-family rental market and potential impacts on renters*. New York: Right to the City Alliance.

Fields, D., & Uffer, S. (2016). The financialisation of rental housing: A comparative analysis of New York City and Berlin. *Urban Studies, 53*(7), 1486–1502.

Grudnoff, M. (2015). *Top gears: How negative gearing and the capital gains tax discount benefit drive up house prices*. Canberra: Australia Institute. https://tinyurl.com/y52x8c82.

Grudnoff, M. (2018). *Who Really Benefits from Negative Gearing?* Canberra: Australia Institute. https://www.tai.org.au/content/who-really-benefits-negative-gearing. Accessed 27 August 2019.

Hulse, K., & Burke, T. (2015). Private rental housing in Australia: Political inertia and market change. In: Dufty Jones, R. & Rogers, D. (eds), *Housing in twenty-first century Australia: People, practices and policies*. London: Routledge.

Hulse, K., & Reynolds, M. (2018). Investification: Financialisation of housing markets and persistence of suburban socio-economic disadvantage. *Urban Studies, 55*(8), 1655–1671.

Hulse, K., Burke, T., Ralston, L., & Stone, W. (2012). *The Australian private rental sector: Changes and challenges* (Positioning Paper 149). Melbourne: AHURI.

Hulse, K., Pawson, H., Reynolds, M., & Herath, S. (2014). *Disadvantaged places in Urban Australia: Analysing Socio-economic Diversity and Housing Market Performance*, No. 225. Melbourne: AHURI.

Hulse, K., Martin, C., James, A., & Stone, W. (2018). *Private rental in transition: institutional change, technology and innovation in Australia*, No. 296. Melbourne: AHURI.

Hulse, K., Reynolds, M., & Martin, C. (2019). The everyman archetype: Discursive reframing of private landlords in the financialization of rental housing. *Housing Studies* (Online First).

Isaac, D. (1998). *Property investment*. London: Palgrave.

Jones Lang LaSalle (JLL). (2019). *Australian student accommodation: investment review & outlook 2019*. Sydney: JLL.

Kemp, P. A. (2015). Private renting after the Global Financial Crisis. *Housing Studies, 30*(4), 601–620.

Lane, I. (2019, February 15). How investors fuelled Australia's historic property boom, *The New Daily*. https://thenewdaily.com.au/finance/property/2019/02/15/why-the-property-bubble-burst/.

Loveridge, S., & Selting, A. C. (1998). A review and comparison of shift-share identities. *International Regional Science Review, 21*(1), 37–58.

Martin, C. (2018). Clever Odysseus: Narratives and strategies of rental property investor subjectivity in Australia. *Housing Studies, 33*(7), 1060–1084.

Mather, J. (2018, January 22). Top 10pc gain 80pc of CGT benefits, *Australian Financial Review*.

Martin, C., Hulse, K., & Pawson, H. (2018). *The changing institutions of private rental housing: An international review*. Final Report No. 292. Melbourne: AHURI.

Parkinson, S., James, A., & Liu, E. (2018). *Navigating a changing private rental sector: Opportunities and challenges for low-income renters* (Final Report No. 302). Melbourne: AHURI.

Pawson, H. (2019). The housing story: An Australian perspective. In: Maclennan, D., Pawson, H., Gibb, K., Chisholm, S. & Hulchanski, D. (eds) *Shaping futures: Changing the housing story*. Glasgow: University of Glasgow.

Pawson, H., & Martin, C. (2020). Rental property investment in disadvantaged areas: The means and motivations of Western Sydney's new landlords. *Housing Studies*. https://doi.org/10.1080/02673037.2019.1709806.

Pawson, H., & Milligan, V. (2013). New dawn or chimera? Can institutional financing transform rental housing? *International Journal of Housing Policy, 13*(4), 335–357.

Pawson, H., Martin, C., van den Nouwelant, R., Milligan, V., Ruming, K., & Melo, M. (2019). *Build-to-rent in Australia: Product feasibility and potential affordable housing contribution*. Sydney: Landcom.

Pawson, H., Milligan, V., & Yates, J. (2020). *Housing policy in Australia: A case for system reform*. Singapore: Palgrave Macmillan.

Randolph, B., & Holloway, D. (2005). The suburbanization of disadvantage in Sydney: New problems new policies. *Opolis, 1*(1), 49–65.

Randolph, B., & Tice, A. (2016). Suburbanizing disadvantage in Australian cities: Sociospatial change in an era of neoliberalism. *Journal of Urban Affairs, 36*(sup1), 384–399.

Rugg, J., & Rhodes, D. (2018). *The evolving private rented sector: Its contribution and potential*. York: University of York.

Scheule, H. (2020, July 31) Why NSW is skewing its tax system toward build-to-rent apartments and away from mum and pop landlords. *The Conversation*. https://theconversation.com/why-nsw-is-skewing-its-tax-system-toward-build-to-rent-apartments-and-away-from-mum-and-pop-landlords-143594.

Seelig, T., Thompson, A., Burke, T., Pinnegar, S., McNelis, S., & Morris, A. (2009). *Understanding what motivates households to become and remain investors in the private rental market*, No. 130. Melbourne: AHURI.

Soaita, A., Searle, B., McKee, K., & Moore, T. (2017). Becoming a landlord: Strategies of property-based welfare in the private rental sector in Britain. *Housing Studies, 32*, 613–637.

Wachsmuth, D., Kerrigan, D., Chaney, D., & Shillolo, A. (2017). *Short-term cities: Airbnb's impact on Canadian housing markets*, Policy report, Urban Politics and Governance research group, School of Urban Planning, McGill University. http://upgo.lab.mcgill.ca/airbnb/.

Wilkins, R. (2016). *The household, income and labour dynamics in Australia survey: Selected findings from waves 1 to 14*. Melbourne: Melbourne Institute.

Wood, G., & Ong, R. (2013). When and why do landlords retain property investments? *Urban Studies, 50*(16), 3243–3261.

Chapter 4
Housing Pathways of Private Renters—Rebounds, Blockages and Dead Ends

Abstract The chapter, drawing on Clapham's concept of housing pathways, examines why people find themselves reliant on the PRS, often for extended periods or even lifelong. Four groups are focused on—long-term renters (ten years or more) who are reliant on the PRS for their accommodation because they have no other option. They are primarily low-income households. The second focus is on older (aged 65 and older) private renters primarily or totally dependent solely on the Age Pension. We then investigate the circumstances of *rentvestors*. These are tenants who cannot afford to buy a home in the area they are currently renting in and have bought a property in a cheaper area. The final group are "choosers"; they have voluntarily decided that renting is a superior option to purchasing. What is apparent is that the primary reason why people find themselves in the PRS for extended periods is because they do not have the financial resources to purchase a home. This was most apparent in the case of tenants reliant on government benefits for their income. However, even households with employed members were locked out of home ownership. In the case of older renters, many had been home owners but primarily because of divorce they lost the family home and found themselves dependent on the PRS. The chapter illustrates that contingency often plays a major role in the housing pathways of individuals. Besides divorce, ill-health, business failure and death of partner can push people out of home ownership into the PRS or, in the case of younger renters, solidify their dependence on the PRS.

Context

In contemporary Australia, just as in comparator countries, there is an increasing division between those who have the resources to choose their housing and lifestyle and those with minimal capacity to do so (Bates et al., 2019; Clapham et al., 2014). As discussed in earlier chapters, growing numbers of Australians are excluded from both home ownership and social housing. The central question examined in this chapter is why are so many Australian households finding themselves reliant on the PRS, often for an extended period or even lifelong? In keeping with previous research, we define long-term renters (LTRs) as those residing in the private rental market for

A. Morris et al., *The Private Rental Sector in Australia*,
https://doi.org/10.1007/978-981-33-6672-5_4

at least ten years. This chapter focuses primarily on the about one in ten Australian households in this situation. Almost all are renting because of limited finances rather than by choice. However, the chapter also profiles a small group who have chosen to be long-term renters.

As discussed in previous chapters a fundamental explanation for PRS growth over recent decades, is the expanding number of aspirant first home buyers barred from home ownership by rising house prices and escalating mortgage loan deposit requirements (Productivity Commission, 2019; Pawson et al., 2020). In a long-term analysis, Yates (2008) showed that the scope for accessing home ownership had declined substantially since the 1970s. This was mainly due to the increasing "deposit gap"—the extra amount a median earner would need to find on top of their maximum allowable loan to afford a typically priced residential property. Thus:

> After some signs of recovery with the decline in interest rates in the mid-1990s, the deposit gap to income ratio is now 3 to 4 times greater than it was in the 1970s, when affordability problems started to emerge. (Yates, 2008, p. 9)

In the decade since Yates's analysis, the deposit gap has continued to increase (Pawson et al., 2020). As discussed in Chapters 1 and 3, the financialisation of housing has meant that in the capital cities, more especially Sydney and Melbourne, residential property prices rocketed during the 2010s, far outstripping wage increases (Jacobs, 2019; Morris, 2018; Hulse et al., 2019). As a result, even allowing for falling interest rates during this period, first home buyer affordability declined significantly. In 2017, economists at the investment bank, UBS, calculated that for the average first time home buyer in Sydney, " … saving a 10% deposit to buy at the average Sydney house price of $1.2 mn would take an incredible 40 years to save" (Haslem et al., 2017).

Barriers to accessing home ownership have been accentuated for many households by the changing nature of Australia's labour force. A sizeable proportion of the labour force are now employed in part-time or casual employment or are under-employed (ABS, 2020; Campbell et al., 2014; Kler et al., 2018). Besides an extremely limited capacity to raise the required deposit, aspirant home buyers in insecure employment are liable to be viewed by mortgage providers as higher risk borrowers and therefore denied access to mortgage finance except at prohibitive rates (Campbell et al., 2014). The economic crisis precipitated by the COVID-19 pandemic has triggered huge job losses which will have exacerbated this situation and generated what are likely to be long-lived impacts (see Borland, 2020).

Another key shift over recent decades has been the nation's changing household composition. In 2016, 24% of households in Australia were single-person households (2.3 million of the 9.2 million households in total), up from 15.7% in 1976 (ABS, 2001, 2017). One-parent families with dependent children constituted 6.5% of all family types in 1976, they now constitute 15% (ABS 2001, 2019a). In 2016 about a quarter of all lone-person households and just under four in ten one-parent families were private renters (Australian Government Productivity Commission, 2019). The capacity of such households to enter (or sustain) home ownership is typically far less than couple households. Thus Hulse et al. (2019, p. 54) show that the majority of Q1 households (the bottom 20% of income earners) in the PRS are lone person households or single parents.

> The biggest groups of Q1 private renter households are single person households of various ages (52 per cent) or single parents with children (22 per cent); relatively low percentages live as a couple (with or without children) or as a group household.

A related significant societal change is the increase in homeowners losing their partner due to divorce or separation. About one in three marriages in Australia end in divorce and a substantial proportion, around 45%, occur after the age of 45 (ABS, 2018). Divorce or separation often has a disruptive impact on housing pathways—often one or both members of a owner-occupier couple that separates falls out of home ownership and becomes dependent on the PRS (Ong et al., 2015; Wiesel, 2014; Wood et al., 2008, 2017). An Australian study drawing on the Housing Income and Labour Dynamics in Australia (HILDA) longitudinal survey[1] established that,

> divorce and separation are a major source of disruption to home ownership aspirations. In a two-year period following household dissolution, rates of home ownership among those who had lost a partner fell from 69 per cent to below 50 per cent. (Wood et al., 2008)

Losing a partner due to bereavement can also have a devastating financial impact and make retaining home ownership difficult (Wood et al., 2017). A major British study[2] found that "Maintaining rent or mortgage payments for a home after the death of a partner was likely to be a major issue for some people ..." (Corden et al., 2008, p. 41).

A final contributory factor to post-1990s PRS growth has been the diminishing capacity of Australia's social housing sector. As discussed in Chapter 1, as a proportion of the national dwelling stock, social housing has declined from 6.2 per 100 households in 1991 to 4.2 in 2018 (Australian Government Productivity Commission, 2019; Pawson et al., 2020). Expressed in terms of annual lettings by public housing agencies and community housing organisations, this trend has been even more stark; using this measure, social housing supply has effectively collapsed by 50% since 1997. As a result, social housing has become extremely difficult to access, even for those on very low incomes and otherwise disadvantaged. For example, in NSW, non-Indigenous older private renters "who have met the normal eligibility criteria for social housing may be approved for housing assistance as an elderly client if they are [a]ged 80 years and over" (NSW Government, 2019).

[1]HILDA is a longitudinal study that has followed the lives of over 17,000 Australians since 2001.

[2]This research drew on 50 in-depth interviews, recruited via the British Household Panel Survey and representative data sets produced by the Office for National Statistics Longitudinal Study.

The "Groups" Focused on and Housing Pathways

The chapter focuses on the trajectory into the formal PRS of four "groups".[3] As stated, the primary focus is on long-term renters (ten years or more) in Sydney and Melbourne who are reliant on the PRS for their accommodation because they have no other option. Many of these households may have entered private rental thinking that it would be transitional, but have then found it difficult or impossible to transition into home ownership or social housing. They are primarily low-income households.

The second focus is older (aged 65 and older) private renters in Sydney and regional NSW mainly or totally reliant on the Age Pension. At present about 7% of Australians aged 65 plus are private tenants (see Table 1.1). These renters are particularly vulnerable as their income is fixed[4] and their capacity to find alternative accommodation is usually extremely limited. Many had rebounded back into the PRS—they had fallen out of home ownership after divorce or another crisis.

The third case study group is tenants who cannot afford to buy a home in their preferred neighbourhood in Sydney or Melbourne and who choose to rent instead in the area in question. These areas are usually well-located in terms of access to high quality schools, transport and other amenities. Within this group a few were *rentvestors*—people renting their own place of residence, while also renting out a property owned elsewhere invariably in a cheaper suburb. This gave them the security of having a stake in the volatile housing market. According to recent research *rentvestors* account for about one in eight private renter households (Hulse & McPherson, 2014).

The final focus is on long-term tenants for whom renting was an active voluntary choice. Although a small proportion, the interviews suggest that households who choose to be long-term renters is a growing phenomenon.

David Clapham's concept of housing pathways is useful for understanding private renters' trajectories. He argues the "housing pathway of a household is the continually changing set of relationships and interactions which it experiences over time in its consumption of housing" (Clapham, 2002, p. 64). Certainly, for many private renters in our research, housing pathways were intimately linked to class origins,

---

[3]The analysis draws mainly on in-depth interviews (see Appendix) conducted with long-term renters in Sydney and Melbourne, Australia's most expensive and populous cities. The interviews were conducted in low, medium and high-rent areas. Interviews were also conducted in Sydney and regional NSW with older (65 plus) private renters reliant on the government Age Pension. Many of these interviewees had recently become dependent on the PRS.

[4]Pensions are means tested and indexed and increased twice a year by the Consumer Price Index (CPI) or Pensioner and Beneficiary Living Cost Index (PBLCI) which ever is the greater. In January 2020, the full government Age Pension was $467 a week for older people living alone and $703.50 a week for couples. Almost all would have been eligible for Rent Assistance (RA). The maximum RA amount in January 2020 was $69.80 a week for people living alone, and $65.80 for couples. The median weekly rent for an apartment in Sydney at the beginning of 2019 was $530 and in Melbourne it was $410 (ABC, https://www.abc.net.au/news/2019-01-10/sydney-house-rent-prices-drop-according-to-domain-data/10704468).

income, education, employment history and relationship or marital status (see Izuhara & Heywood, 2003). Interviewees who lived alone and divorced or single parents, usually had limited financial resources and few housing options. Clapham goes on to argue that "a housing pathway will run alongside and be closely associated with other types of pathways such as employment" (2002, p. 65). The housing pathways of renters reliant on government benefits or in irregular casual employment, would have severely restricted housing options in expensive housing markets like Sydney and Melbourne. However, according to our evidence, even some of those in well-paid jobs were constrained with respect to housing options. As discussed below, while potentially able to rent in well-located neighbourhoods, local house purchase was often out of reach for this cohort.

In sum, for many interviewees a key reason for renting was the simple impossibility of home ownership due to the financial constraint of being confined to low-income employment or benefit reliance. For others, divorce or separation in the context of traditional gender roles and employment histories was a key factor. Other cited reasons included falling out with children, disruption in income due to retrenchment, poor health or death of a spouse and being unable to access social housing. These factors are discussed in turn. The decision by more affluent households to rent in areas where ownership is unaffordable, is then discussed. The chapter concludes with an examination of individuals / households who have chosen to rent long-term.

Priced Out of Home Ownership

As discussed in prior chapters the increasing financialisation of housing in Melbourne and Sydney, has led to massive price increases in residential property since the turn of the century[5] (Aalbers, 2016; Morris, 2018, 2021; Pawson et al., 2020). In relation to local incomes, both cities are amongst the most expensive globally and similar to other cities with expensive residential real estate, people's capacity to purchase a home is often dependent on a dual income and/or substantial assistance from family (see Core Data, 2019; Lennartz & Ronald, 2018). Not surprisingly the interviews indicated that the incapacity to purchase a home was especially true of single adults (with or without children) and those in low-paid employment or reliant on welfare benefits. Naturally, renters in well-paid jobs tended to be more optimistic about their future housing prospects, with many anticipating future home ownership.

Albeit not confined to long-term renters, results from our survey in Sydney and Melbourne[6] were consistent with in-depth interview findings. Thus, only 44% of respondents reliant on government benefits ($n = 70$) agreed or strongly agreed that

[5]In June 2019, the median house price in Sydney was $875,000 and in Melbourne it was $680,000. Banks generally require at least a 10% deposit (i.e. $87,500 in Sydney and $68,000 in Melbourne at this time). In May 2019, the average full-time earnings in NSW was $86,372 per annum and in Victoria it was $83,616 (ABS 2019b).

[6]Our renters survey, undertaken in 2015 in high-rent (inner city), medium-rent (middle suburb) and low-rent (outer suburb) areas of Sydney and Melbourne involved 600 face-to-face interviews

they expected to own their home in retirement; in contrast, 80% of respondents whose income was a wage or salary ($n = 443$) expected to do so. About 12% of the latter group, already owned a home elsewhere. Lone person households and single parents were significantly less likely than couples (with or without children) to anticipate having transitioned to home ownership by the end of their working lives. Only 45% of the former grouping agreed or strongly agreed that they expected to own a place by the time they retired verse 79% of couple households.

Catherine (mid-forties, all the names used are pseudonyms) lived by herself in a low-rent area in outer Melbourne. She had no illusions about her situation: "I'll be renting for the rest of my life unless I find a partner who is rich and has a house already." Rodney (33) lived by himself in Sydney's outer suburbs. He had a scrappy employment history and at the time of the interview was on a Disability Support Pension (DSP)[7] having suffered a work-injury. He foresaw no possibility of home ownership.

> I've always struggled with work and I was on a disability pension even before I hurt my back … Just some psychological problem … Always managed them, always tried to get work and keep work. It's just that I hurt myself also. Got a massive back injury to go with it [mental health issues] about six years ago and that just made things even more difficult for me, so renting is the only option for me at the moment.

Mark (72) had never married and had always been in low paying jobs:

> I would have liked to have owned my own house naturally, but I've never been able to sort of save up enough money. I've always been sort of battling and struggling on. I couldn't get any education at all because mum was on her own and she was struggling really bad, so as soon as I turned 15, I was virtually out of school to get a job … So I've virtually never been able to save enough money to buy a house.

Tracey (early forties), a single parent with three children in a low-rent area in Sydney, had been renting for 21 years. Asked why she had remained in rental housing, she responded:

> A lack of financial savvy to have gotten a deposit together in my 20s and I did a bit of a dance on my credit rating … I'm never going to own property which is heartbreaking now I've gotten older and I realise what that means. It's terrible, but it is where I'm at. I'm not in a position where I think I'll ever be able to buy a home.

Child-care responsibilities meant that Tracey had only worked intermittently: "And I've been at home with the kids for a lot of years, so my financial status isn't good in that sense you know. I'm not an income earner or anything like that".

Stephanie was also a single parent in Sydney's low-rent outer suburbs:

> I don't really have the money to be able to buy my own property and with buying your own property comes a lot of hassles, land rates and everything else that goes on top of it, your bills everything. And my bills are pretty high on their own and being on a single parent pension, his father doesn't give me crap, he takes more than he gives, so I just can't afford it.

---

with private tenants identified from tenancy bond lodgement records. For a full account of the methodology see Appendix.

[7]In April 2020 the Disability Support Pension (DSP) for sole person households was $463 a week. This excludes Rent Assistance.

The inability to save the requisite mortgage deposit was not only a problem faced by sole person households, but was also experienced by some couples. Jean and her husband (low-rent Sydney) had constantly struggled financially and could not look to other family members for help:

> Well we never sort of managed to get enough for a deposit on a house or anything like that. We had six children and by the time you look after them, there wasn't any [money] left.

When Maria and Noel, a couple in their mid-thirties who were both employed and renting in a high-rent area in Sydney, were asked whether they expected to be long-term renters, Maria responded:

> You're trying to save up the deposit … and they [house prices] keep increasing and you sort of miss the opportunities sometimes. And it is like now it is just beyond our scope to even get a place because the deposit and million dollar house and apartments, we just can't afford it … Yeah, I really regret that we [didn't] … put in an offer.

A few interviewees spoke about having narrowly missed out on property acquisition earlier in their lives, a prospect now seemingly ruled out by subsequent house price inflation. Emily, early forties, had considered buying in Melbourne, but was now resigned to a lifetime of renting:

> I thought of it [buying a property] a few times … In hindsight, it's probably a shame I didn't because they were affordable then. Even though they still seemed expensive, but now it's just off the Richter scale, especially if you want somewhere that's still close to the city … I've given up now. There's no way now. The prices have just gone ridiculous.

Extended family commitments made it difficult for Abahd (high-rent area in Melbourne) to save for a deposit. He was supporting his family in Bangladesh:

> Yeah, well one day, I'm hoping [to buy a house]. As I said, we are saving up … I do tend to send money overseas as well to help my family members, so it becomes a bit challenging … and there's a lot of stuff on your plate and you've got to manage everything.

Disruption in Income and Accumulation of Disadvantage

Bates et al., (2019) in their study of older people in New Zealand, highlight how misfortune can result in households rapidly finding themselves in a precarious housing situation. For some of our interviewees disruption of income due to divorce /separation, retrenchment, poor health or death of spouse had played a central role in their housing trajectory (see Wood et al., 2017). It catapulted them into a precarious position which led to a loss of the family home which they had owned, or alternatively increased the likelihood of lifelong renting. Not surprisingly, low-income households tended to be more vulnerable to critical events as Stone et al. (2015, p. 2) conclude in their study on sustaining private rental tenancies:

> The impact of lost income capacity resulting from some critical life events is more pronounced among low to moderate income private renters than medium or high-income private renters.

Divorce and Separation

Divorce or separation was a central reason for interviewees, especially older women, finding themselves dependent on the PRS. Many of our older research participants had been home owners, however divorce had catapulted them into the PRS. Drawing on the HILDA survey of Australian households, Wood et al. (2008, p. 1), found that dissolution of relationships had a serious impact on housing affordability for just under a third of the couples involved:

> One year following dissolution, 30.7 per cent of the sample moved into housing affordability stress (HAS) (paying more than 30 per cent of income in housing costs), compared to 8.9 per cent of the sample who experienced HAS in the year preceding household dissolution.

Almost all of our older (65 plus) female interviewees had been in marriages characterised by traditional gender roles, thus many had little in the way of a formal employment history, having devoted their married lives primarily to child-rearing. After divorce, most found it extremely difficult to secure work that would allow them to retain or regain home ownership. Reduced income forced them into the PRS. Many were desperately endeavouring to access social housing. Having rarely had paid work during her marriage, Barbara (70) had accrued little superannuation. She saw her situation as very much a gender issue:

> I had $6,000 [superannuation] because in my era women didn't work. Men didn't want their women to work, so you stayed at home and reared the children, and there was no such thing as superannuation. And as you got older, you went on the pension. Everybody did, you know. And of course, then it changed, but I was then in my fifties and so for me, I sort of fell through the cracks.

The housing pathway of Harriet (66) was similar:

> When I was married we had our own home. After the divorce, I couldn't afford one. I was also you know, well over 50 … I had been retired from the workforce for quite a number of years before the marriage broke down and I had to rent. I didn't have a recent employment history, so it took me quite a while to find some sort of work.

Divorce could also have disastrous implications for older men. Steve (66), a former homeowner, had been renting for several years after the breakdown of his marriage:

> I mean I've been renting for seven years, eight years, ever since my wife threw me out … I mean we used to own our own home … Well I was well into my 30s before I got married and I was married for 22 or 23 years. And she gave me the flick. And took just about everything. But I agreed to it basically because at that stage with a twelve-year-old daughter … But I basically allowed her to take what she'd got from the house so that she could look after Samantha.

Gary had also been a homeowner and lost the family home after his divorce:

> Well, I did have my own house, but the divorce took everything and so that's the situation. It wasn't planned and then I hadn't been able to get back into the market again. So, it was a bad decision on my behalf there. You can't predict the future.

Some of the younger interviewees had also been severely affected by divorce. Cassandra, in her forties, had been a home owner in an expensive Sydney suburb prior to the dissolution of her marriage. After subsequently renting in a high rent neighbourhood in Sydney for 11 years she had been unable to accumulate sufficient savings for a mortgage deposit:

> Well we divorced and then there was a settlement. We'd been in quite a valuable house … and I got paid out of that … My daughter was a baby and so I was looking at a long period of not being able to work very much. And so you know at the time it seemed sensible to … invest that money and to live off some returns off it and work a little bit and rent …

Most of the younger interviewees who had divorced or separated, had been renting at that time. Rather than being forced out of home ownership, the experience had deepened their financial vulnerability and dependence on renting. Prior to her divorce Louise (early 40s in high-rent area in Sydney) and her ex-husband had been actively saving for a deposit. However, divorce had entrenched her private rental status:

> We were at the stage where we were going to be putting money away for a deposit to buy somewhere and then it [the marriage] all went wrong, so that was that … And even if we had been homeowners … in separating we would have had to sell and then we both would have ended up renting anyway you know because I couldn't have sustained a mortgage … with my salary at the time having a small child … You know you've got a good job that pays pretty well, but I was working you know part-time and I had a child in child-care which was then $85 a day … So you know, there's things like that, that preclude people you know paying a massive mortgage.

Retrenchment, Bankruptcy, Poor Health, Death of Partner

Disruption of income due to retrenchment, business collapse, poor health or death of spouse could lead to a loss of the family home and dependence on the PRS. For Ron (68) a particularly bad period in his life had resulted in the loss of the family home. Although able to find work after a period of unemployment, poor health truncated his working life and he was never able to accrue enough capital to regain home ownership:

> We did own a home briefly when we lived in Sydney, but I had some issues with both drinking and gambling and that caused a change of jobs and we moved to the South Coast back in 1996 ... and initially lived in a caravan while I searched for work. So that period was … fairly bad … for us. But about 1998 … I was lucky to get a very good job with a company in Sydney … Yeah, so that allowed us to build up some finances again, but not to the extent where we thought we could probably buy a place and still have some money left over and that's how we found ourselves [in private rental] and I finished up having a minor heart attack in October 2010 … so consequently I stopped work and yeah, hadn't, as I said, built up my finances nearly as much as we'd liked to be able to buy a place.

Michaela recounted how she and her ex-husband lost their home due to business bankruptcy. Soon afterwards the marriage collapsed:

> We lost the house. The bank took the house. He bought a business and it went into debt so the bank took the house to cover the money for the business. Things just went completely kaput. I went my way with my kids. He went his way … So basically I moved along. I always rented. I couldn't get finance to purchase a home for myself in those days, even though I was working.

The death of a spouse can have dramatic financial implications and lead to the surviving partner having to exit home ownership (see Cordon et al., 2008; Wood et al., 2017). Kate (72) and her husband, former homeowners, had sold up and moved into the hotel business. They lived in the hotels they leased. After her husband's passing, private rental was Kate's only option. Asked whether she ever expected to find herself renting in the private market, Kate responded:

> No, I never ever thought I would. …When my husband died that was just such a shock. … I often regret selling the home that we had … He thought we were doing the best and at that stage of the game we never ever thought that he was going to you know have coronaries and things like that …

Isobel (73) had been a homeowner in an affluent suburb in Sydney her whole married life. She lost the family home after her husband died leaving massive debts:

> My husband died 10 years … and really I mean, I was very lucky. I'd a lot of good friends and friends stood by me … But that's the reason [I'm in private rental] and it's always been very foreign to me. As soon as we could we went out and bought and I never wanted to rent in my life, but I hadn't got the choice, yeah.

Fall out with Children

Although there are no specific statistics on its prevalence in Australia, studies in Canada and the United Kingdom concluded that two to eight per cent of people aged 65 and over experience at least one form of abuse annually and that it is mostly intra-familial and intergenerational in nature (Australian Government, 2019). For a few of our older adult interviewees their move into the PRS had been precipitated by a dispute with a son or daughter. Carol's (67, low-rent, Sydney) account was particularly poignant. She had been a private renter for only five months when interviewed, having previously lived with her daughter and son-in-law for over a decade:

> My daughter [and I] bought a house together before she got married, and … she kicked me out … I lived with my daughter and her three kids and husband … She promised to never to kick me out of the house … and that I'd be there forever, and I looked after the kids for 10 years and then her husband decided that I was not welcome.

An elderly couple had been forced to sell their home and move into the PRS after their daughter, having met a new partner, claimed a share of their house. Legal action had failed to prevent the loss of their home:

> My daughter … had moved jobs and was a bit desperate for money on her own with three children, so we moved into the granny flat and gave her the house. Then the boyfriend came along and they decided that they wanted a share of the house, so we were forced to sell. It

> was a terrible two years for us. We had to go to court and everything cost us over $400,000 in fees and such like and that was money we didn't really have ... I [have] just turned 77 and my husband's 80, so to have your daughter stab you in the back you know, it was dreadful. (Cherie)

An Inability to Access Social Housing

For some interviewees, despite being eligible to register for social housing, the severe shortage made ongoing reliance on the PRS unavoidable. Douglas (72) had found himself locked out of social housing:

> I've been on a list now for about seven years and I'm still waiting .... The last time I was out there they were telling me about ten years. I tried to put my name down [for social housing] before I retired and I had to take them in a statement about how much money I was earning, and they said, "No, you cannot get on the Department of Housing list because you're earning too much money." I said, "I want to put my name down now, so that I can have a house when I retire because when I retire I won't be able to [afford to rent] ... And they said, "No. There's nothing we can do about that. That's a government rule".

When Pamela (68) inquired about accessing social housing at the age of 71, she was told, "Come back when you're 80". In NSW people reliant on the government Age Pension, "may be approved for housing assistance as an elderly client" only when they turn eighty and if they are Indigenous Australians, when they turn 55 (NSW Government, 2006).

After leaving the family home, Carol battled to find a place to rent and was forced to move into a refuge for homeless women for a few weeks. She had tried to obtain social housing, but was rebuffed:

> I went to the Department of Housing and they keep promising. They keep saying they are going to put me on the priority list[8] and then when I go up there next time they said that I'm not priority. I'm not on priority list and that I had to find myself a private rental, that I may wait to the extent of 15 years to get a place [in social housing].

Barbara (70) was desperate to access social housing: "It's [being a private renter] eating into any bit of capital I have, and I have put my name down for public housing. I've been accepted for public housing [she was eligible to be on the public housing waiting-list], but of course the waiting-list is huge".[9]

---

[8] In NSW the waiting list for social housing is divided into a priority and general waiting list. If a person is placed on the priority waiting list, the waiting period is shorter. Nationally, in 2017–2018 "among new allocations to greater needs households, 73% or 11,400 received public housing within one year of the household being on the waiting list" (AIHW 2019). In NSW, at the end of June 2019, there were 46,530 applicants on the general waiting list and 4,484 were on the "priority" list (NSW Government, 2020). Nationally, if placed on the general waiting list, the wait could be up to ten years or even longer and as a consequence many people do not bother to apply (Productivity Commission, 2019, p. 25).

[9] Barbara eventually accessed social housing about seven years after being interviewed.

Homeownership Aspirations, But Unable to Purchase in Desired Area

The desire to live in a well-located and resourced area with good public [government] schools was an important consideration for several interviewees especially in the high-rent areas. While home ownership was ideally desired, it had been traded off for residing in a convenient location brimming with amenities, but where the cost of housing was prohibitive (see Hulse & McPherson, 2014). Noteworthy, is that 9% of respondents to our survey were *rentvestors*—they owned a residential property elsewhere. Not surprisingly they were overwhelmingly located in the high and medium rent areas. Only 2.5% of the respondents in low-rent areas had a residential property elsewhere, compared to 16.5% in high-rent and 8.5% in medium-rent areas.

Graham, his partner and teenage daughter lived in a high-rent area in Sydney. They could not contemplate buying in the area, but were attracted by its convenient location and by their daughter's high quality public school. They had purchased a property in an affordable area about 80 kms north of Sydney where they planned to retire:

> Yeah, well the main reason was my daughter goes to Mosman High and she can walk to Mosman High from here and there's also you know with schools there's a catchment area so you have to be in a certain area to go to the school, so that's one of the reasons why … We can afford to rent here, but we can't afford to buy here, so that's the pay off. We were thinking of retiring down the coast, so we actually bought an investment property for … like $300,000 as opposed to, you can't get a shoe box for $300,000 in Sydney. It is just ridiculous …

Access to high quality public schooling was also a key factor for Rachel, a mother of four school-going children in a high-rent area of inner-Melbourne:

> There's a good high school here. We wanted to get into the local area, so we could attend there. That's the main reason [we moved here]. That is the reason.

Although Brooke and her husband earned well, they could not afford to buy in the high-rent area in Sydney they resided in. The location (close to the city and the beach), high quality amenities and the schools were key drawcards.:

> Sure it [home ownership] provides you with security and you don't have that stress of … having to move. I get that, but at the same time you know for us, for example, if we wanted to buy we'd be paying four times what we pay at the moment in a mortgage … It doesn't really make financial sense to go and do that … You have to live somewhere. So I choose to live in a nice area where my children are [at school] …

Living by oneself made it all the more difficult to purchase. Liz, mid-forties, wanted to purchase a property, but could not afford to buy in her upmarket high-rent Sydney locality:

> It's [the area] very nice and that's the main reason I've stayed here for so long. Obviously I'd like to [purchase] a property]. You know ideally I'd like to live in Mosman, but in my own property, but I sort of didn't really strike at the right time and so now the prices are so ridiculous.

Mel was living by herself in a high-rent area in inner Melbourne. She had a similar narrative to Liz and was thinking of becoming a *rentvestor*.

> I probably realistically won't be able to afford to buy where I want to live … I probably will stay renting in North Melbourne, but I wouldn't mind getting a house or something … So I would like to own something … Like I know people who have moved out to the sticks because it's the only place they can afford to buy a house. And that's fine, if that's the only place I can afford to buy a house, I'll buy a house there … I would never live there … No, I would continue to rent somewhere that I wanted to live.

Choosing to Rent

As argued in Chapter 2, Australia's private rental regulation remains weighted towards landlord interests and—by the standards of at least some comparator countries—provides tenants with relatively weak legal rights and protection. Actively choosing to rent under such conditions may appear unlikely. However, for some renters personal circumstances and life-style preferences mean that renting is viewed positively. It may even extend beyond this—as an active rejection of home ownership as a culturally-sanctioned ideal. As Brown and Vergragt (2016, p. 313) conclude in their discussion on contemporary urban millennials, they will "very likely have to redefine their aspirations for good life in a way that does not depend on amassing material possessions and consumerism". The flexibility of the PRS was especially appreciated by "choosers". They considered that renting conferred the freedom to move or travel when desired. Bauman's concept of liquid modernity highlights the increasing desire for transience in the contemporary (albeit pre-COVID-19) period:

> Transience has replaced durability at the top of the value table. What is valued today (by choice as much as by unchosen necessity) is the ability to be on the move, to travel light and at short notice. Power is measured by the speed with which responsibilities can be escaped. Who accelerates, wins; who stays put, loses. (Bauman & Tester, 2001, p. 95)

Most of the choosers interviewed in our research were single, financially comfortable and living in highly desirable high-rent areas of Sydney or Melbourne. The flexibility that private renting offered was generally the primary motivation. Since moving to Australia in the mid-1970s, Kim (Melbourne, high-rent area) had always rented: "Well since I came to Australia in 1977, I rented. I didn't want to buy. Got close [to buying] a couple of times, but changed my mind". She loved travelling, so the flexibility that renting provided was viewed as a major advantage:

> I just travel anywhere and everywhere. I thought no, and if you've got a house you're stuck there, and I thought, no. I work hard for my money, so that money that I work hard for is for me not to have a [permanent] roof over my head. As long as I've got food in my mouth and clothing on my back ... Renting has been good for me because I can still do what I want.

Myra lived in a studio apartment in a high-rent area in Sydney and had no intention of ever purchasing a home. She had moved to Sydney from Europe 20 years prior, was single, in her late thirties, earned well and enjoyed the flexibility that renting accorded.

Also, she viewed not having to worry about the housing market and maintenance as key advantages. The possibility of being asked to vacate did not bother her:

> I guess that I could pack up and go. I don't have to worry about mortgage, about selling the place. I don't have to worry about the market being really bad, … You know, I don't have to worry about anything. And yeah … and if they should say, "Look we're selling, you have to move out", I know that I can always move in with a friend until I find something, so yeah.

In Melbourne, Leanne inherited a third of a house, but rather than using the proceeds to buy a property, she had decided to continue renting in a high-rent inner suburb where she had lived ever since her divorce 30 years prior:

> I also decided I'd rather travel because I used to [travel and] loved travelling before I had children, and living overseas and things. So I thought rather than put their money into a house, which was my third of my parents' estate at that stage, I would invest it and I could travel and go to concerts and live the life I wanted to lead, so that's basically what I did and I'm still renting.

She felt secure in her accommodation and was confident that her economic and social capital would ensure that she would always have a place to stay:

> Well I'm aware they could ask me to move, and then I would have to find somewhere else. I also know I've got friends. I'd be able to find somewhere else. I wouldn't be homeless.

One of the few families that had made a decision to rent rather than buy, was Suzanne. She lived with her partner and young child in an inner-city area in Melbourne. Her personal history had encouraged a view that renting is advantageous:

> Maybe because I've always rented, I feel like this is like the way that we live normal like … We rent because we've sort of chosen to … and I think that does come back to that I don't think that there's anything wrong with renting because my parents were renters and … we were okay.

Some interviewees revealed more unusual and less positive reasons for deciding to rent. Rosemary (low-rent area, Sydney) was concerned about the future of her relationship and felt that her situation required the flexibility associated with renting:

> Well with my ex, I'll say husband, cos we were together for seven years, the relationship was rocky and you can't predict the future, but I knew it wasn't going to end up in marriage and kids and all that kind of crap … We were both working, both earning good money and we could have afforded to buy a house between us … but for me, it was like no. I don't know where this is going, so no way. I'm not going to put myself in that predicament [having a joint mortgage] and then have to go through court to go, "This is mine, this is yours", all that crap. But so it was my choice to rent and to stick to it … I'm not going to rely on anybody else for anything, no way.

Her renter status allowed her to make a rapid, clean break with her partner:

> I just got up one day and walked cos I knew he was going to ask me to marry him the next day, so I said, "I'm just going to go to the shops to get a packet of cigarettes". I left everything behind. I went for a walk, never went home.

Conclusion

Clearly every trajectory into the PRS is unique, as are the possibilities for moving out and rebounding back again. However, our interview evidence highlights some common themes. Relatively few people are long-term renters by choice, although such a cohort does exist in contemporary Sydney and Melbourne. Most would prefer home ownership or, especially in the case of the older private renters, social housing. Whereas most of the low-income renters were resigned to perpetual renting, many tenants renting in more expensive areas remained confident of accessing homeownership by the time they retired.

Noteworthy, is the role of relationship breakdown. For many of the interviewees divorce or separation had cemented their private rental status. Marriage dissolution also resulted in rebounds—people losing the family home and finding themselves in the PRS either immediately or after a period of time. As mentioned, a number of the older renters had been home owners when married. Besides marital breakdown, ill-health, business failure, retrenchment and the death of a spouse led to interviewees losing their owned home. Often these causes over-lapped. Thus business failure would precipitate divorce and or poor health. Perhaps the saddest situations were those involving older tenants forced out of home ownership after a fall-out with a son or daughter. Evicted, they found themselves in desperate straits in unfamiliar territory. Sadly, many of the older interviewees were desperate to access social housing, but due to the desperate shortage and resultant tight eligibility criteria it was not possible.

Another group focused on were those renters in expensive areas who could afford to buy, but not in the area they were renting in at present. They were keen to stay in the area they were currently residing in, due to the convenient location and high quality schools and amenities. A small proportion were *rentvestors*—tenants owning a rental dwelling elsewhere. It is likely that continuing increases in house prices in the inner-ring in Sydney and Melbourne will result in *rentvestors* becoming a more common phenomenon.

The final focus was on *choosers*—tenants who were renting by choice for the long-term. Although limited in number, this lifestyle choice may be becoming more common. For choosers the flexibility of the PRS is viewed as liberating. Home ownership is viewed as a burden that ties one down. For many choosers, their decision is made much easier by the knowledge that they have the resources to find alternative rental accommodation or can rely on family or friends for a period if they have to move. They have the economic and social capital to cope. Also, most had no dependents so moving was relatively easy.

References

Aalbers, M. B. (2016). *The financialisation of housing: A political economy approach.* Abingdon: Routledge.

ABS (Australian Bureau of Statistics). (2001). *1301.0—Year book Australia, 2001, A century of population change in Australia.* Canberra, ACT: Australian Bureau of Statistics. https://www.abs.gov.au/Ausstats/abs@.nsf/Lookup/0B82C2F2654C3694CA2569DE002139D9.

ABS (Australian Bureau of Statistics). (2017). *2071.0—Census of population and housing: Reflecting Australia—stories from the census.* Canberra: ABS.

ABS (Australian Bureau of Statistics). (2018). *3310.0—Marriages and divorces, Australia, 2017.* Canberra, ACT: Australian Bureau of Statistics. https://www.abs.gov.au/ausstats/abs@.nsf/Latestproducts/3310.0Main%20Features42017?opendocument&tabname=Summary&prodno=3310.0&issue=2017&num=&view=.

ABS (Australian Bureau of Statistics). (2019a, June). *6224.0.55.001—Labour force, Australia: labour force status and other characteristics of families.* Canberra, ACT: Australian Bureau of Statistics. https://www.abs.gov.au/ausstats/abs@.nsf/mf/6224.0.55.001.

ABS (Australian Bureau of Statistics). (2019b, May). *6302.0 Average weekly earnings, Australia.* Canberra, ACT: Australian Bureau of Statistics. https://www.abs.gov.au/ausstats/abs%40.nsf/mediareleasesbyCatalogue/030E8BEF4B0B915ECA2582EA00193B04?OpenDocument.

ABS (Australian Bureau of Statistics). (2020). *6202.0 Labour force, Australia, Dec 2019.* Canberra, ACT: Australian Bureau of Statistics. https://www.abs.gov.au/ausstats/abs@.nsf/mf/6202.0.

AHURI (Australian Housing and Urban Research Institute). (2017). *Census data shows falling proportion of households in social housing.* AHURI (Australian Housing and Urban Research Institute). https://www.ahuri.edu.au/policy/ahuri-briefs/census-shows-falling-proportion-of-households-in-social-housing .

AIHW (Australian Institute of Health and Welfare) . (2019). *Housing assistance in Australia.* Canberra, ACT: Australian Government.

Australian Government. (2019). *Protecting the rights of older Australians.* Canberra, ACT: Attorney Generals Department. https://www.ag.gov.au/RightsAndProtections/protecting-the-rights-of-older-australians/Pages/default.aspx.

Australian Institute of Family Studies. (2017). *Population and households.* Canberra, ACT: Australian Institute of Family Studies, Australian Government. https://aifs.gov.au/facts-and-figures/population-and-households.

Bates, L., Kearns, R., Coleman, T., & Wiles, J. (2019). 'You can't put your roots down': Housing pathways, rental tenure and precarity in older age. *Housing Studies.* https://doi.org/10.1080/02673037.2019.1673323.

Bauman, Z., & Tester, K. (2001). *Conversations with Zygmunt Bauman.* Cambridge: Polity.

Borland, J. (2020). *Labour market snapshot #60: COVID-19 and the Australian labour market: What do the data tell us happened between March and April?* Melbourne, VIC: Department of Economics, University of Melbourne.

Brown, H. S., & Vergragt, P. J. (2016). From consumerism to wellbeing: Toward a cultural transition? *Journal of Cleaner Production, 132,* 308–317.

Campbell, I., Parkinson, S. & Wood, G. (2014). *Underemployment and housing insecurity: An empirical analysis of hILDA Data, No. 230.* Melbourne, VIC: AHURI (Australian Housing and Urban Research Institute).

Clapham, D. (2002). Housing pathways: A post modern analytical framework. *Housing, Theory and Society, 19*(2), 57–68.

Clapham, D., Mackie, P., Orford, S., Thomas, I., & Buckley, K. (2014). The housing pathways of young people in the UK. *Environment and Planning A: Economy and Space, 46*(8), 2016–2031.

Corden, A., Hirst, M. & Nice, K. (2008). *Financial implications of death of a partner* (Working Paper No. ESRC 2288 12.08). York: Social Policy Research Unit, University of York. https://www.york.ac.uk/inst/spru/research/pdf/Bereavement.pdf.

Core Data. (2019). *The Genworth first home buyers sentiment report*. Sydney, NSW: Genworth. https://www.genworth.com.au/media/2030/201909-genworth-fhb-whitepaper-v60.pdf.

Haslem, S., Tharenu, G., & Xu, J. (2017). *Australian economic perspectives: Are first home buyers locked out of housing?* Sydney, NSW: UBS, Global Research. https://neo.ubs.com/shared/d1ZatPa3iM8ech/.

Hulse, K., & McPherson, A. (2014). Exploring dual housing tenure status as a household response to demographic, social and economic change. *Housing Studies, 29*(8), 1028–1044.

Hulse, K., Reynolds, M., Nygaard, C., Parkinson, S. & Yates, J. (2019) *The supply of affordable private rental housing in Australian cities: Short-term and longer-term changes*. Melbourne, VIC: AHURI (Australian Housing and Urban Research Institute). https://www.ahuri.edu.au/research/final-reports/323, https://doi.org/10.18408/ahuri-5120101.

Izuhara, M., & Heywood, F. (2003). A lifetime of inequality: A structural analysis of housing careers and issues facing older private tenants. *Ageing & Society, 23*, 207–224.

Jacobs, K. (2019). *Neoliberal housing policy: An international perspective*. Routledge: London.

Kler, P., Hussain, A., & Shankar, S. (2018). Underemployment in Australia: A panel investigation. *Applied Economics Letters, 25*(1), 24–28.

Lennartz, C., & Ronald, R. (2018). Introduction to the special issue 'housing careers, intergenerational support and family relations.' *Housing Studies, 33*(2), 147–159. https://doi.org/10.1080/02673037.2017.1416070.

Morris, A. (2018). The financialisation of housing and the housing affordability crisis in Sydney. *Housing Finance International, XXXI, 1*(4), 63–69.

Morris, A. (2021). An impossible task? Neoliberalism, the financialistion of housing and the City of Sydney's endeavours to address its housing affordability crisis, *International Journal of Housing Policy, 21*(1), 23–47.

NSW Government. (2006). *Eligibility for social housing entitlements*. Sydney: Communities & Justice, NSW Government. https://www.facs.nsw.gov.au/housing/policies/social-housing-eligibility-allocations-policy-supplement/chapters/entitlements#age.

NSW Government. (2019). *Social housing eligibility and allocations policy supplement*. Sydney, NSW: Communities and Justice, NSW Government. https://www.facs.nsw.gov.au/housing/policies/social-housing-eligibility-allocations-policy-supplement/chapters/entitlements.

NSW Government. (2020). *Applicants on the NSW social housing register at 30 June 2019: Social housing eligibility and allocations policy supplement*. Sydney, NSW: Communities and Justice, NSW Government. https://www.facs.nsw.gov.au/housing/help/applying-assistance/expected-waiting-times.

Ong, R., Wood, G., & Colic-Peisker, V. (2015). Housing older Australians: Loss of homeownership and pathways into housing assistance. *Urban Studies, 52*(16), 2979–3000.

Pawson, H., Milligan, V., & Yates, J. (2020). *Housing policy in Australia: A case for system reform*. London: Palgrave Macmillan.

Productivity Commission. (2019). *Vulnerable private renters; Evidence and options*. Canberra, ACT: Australian Government.

Stone, W., Sharam, A., Wiesel, I., Ralston, L., Markkanen, S. & James, A. (2015). *Accessing and sustaining private rental tenancies: Critical life events, housing shocks and insurances*. Melbourne: AHURI (Australian Housing and Urban Research Institute).

Wiesel, I. (2014). Mobilities of disadvantage: The housing pathways of low-income Australians. *Urban Studies, 51*(2), 319–334.

Wood, G. A., Chamberlain, C., Babbacan, A., Dockery, M., Cullen, G., Costello, G., Nygaard, A., Stoakes A., Adam, M. & Moloney, K. (2008). *The implications of loss of a partner for older private renters* (Final Report No. 116). Melbourne, VIC: AHURI (Australian Housing and Urban Research Institute).

Wood, G. A., Smith, S. J., Cigdem, M., & Ong, R. (2017). Life on the edge: A perspective on precarious home ownership in Australia and the UK. *International Journal of Housing Policy, 17*(2), 201–226.

Yates, J. (2008). *Affordability and access to home ownership: past, present and future? National Research Venture 3: Housing affordability for lower income Australians* (Research Report No. 10). Melbourne, VIC: AHURI (Australian Housing and Urban Research Institute).

Chapter 5
Finding a Rental Property and Feeling at Home

Abstract This chapter examines the process of finding rented accommodation, whether tenants feel at home in their accommodation and what contributes or detracts from a sense of home. The capacity to secure a suitable rental property varies dramatically and is shaped fundamentally by a tenants' financial resources. The massive shortage of affordable rentals for low-income households makes securing suitable accommodation for this group exceptionally difficult and extremely stressful. Single parents, people reliant on government benefits and older renters found securing suitable accommodation particularly hard. Often their only option was to accept rundown properties in the outer suburbs, in areas with few services or amenities. Some renters were forced to leave the metropolitan area so as to find affordable accommodation. Once accommodation was secured, most tenants were able to create a sense of home. The capacity to feel at home was shaped by the condition of the dwelling, the landlord's willingness to do necessary repairs and the tenant–landlord/real estate agent relationship. When tenants had a sound relationship with their landlord or real estate agent they felt secure. The capacity to personalise the space was also an important contributor to feeling at home. For some tenants, the convenience of the neighbourhood and close social ties with neighbours played an important role in them feeling at home.

Introduction

This chapter examines the challenges renters face finding accommodation and their ability to create a sense of home in their rented property. Investigating whether private renters are able to feel at home involves probing issues around landlord-tenant relations, maintenance, the condition and suitability of the accommodation, and the impact of restrictions, for example around keeping pets.

Research around finding a rental property is surprisingly scant. Most work in this area has focused on issues of discrimination and has shown that physical characteristics, religion and ethnic origin can significantly influence the decisions of landlords or real estate agents (Heylen & Van den Broeck, 2016; MacDonald et al., 2016). In Australia, studies have revealed that people with a disability, Indigenous

A. Morris et al., *The Private Rental Sector in Australia*,
https://doi.org/10.1007/978-981-33-6672-5_5

Australians, Muslims and people from India, experience prejudice in the rental market (MacDonald et al., 2016; Victorian Equal Opportunity and Human Rights Commission, 2012; Soatia et al., 2020). A Sydney study using a mystery shopping approach adapted from the USA (people of different backgrounds masquerading as prospective tenants), found "that Anglo testers were treated significantly more favourably than minority testers on several meaningful dimensions that may be expected to impact upon rental housing search experiences" (MacDonald et al., 2016, p. 381).

Compared to homeowners and social housing tenants, moving house is a relatively common phenomenon for private renters in Australia. A study by Stone et al. (2013) drawing on ABS data established that 39.5% of renters had moved three or more times in the last five years, compared to 7.8% of households in other tenures. Just over four in ten private renters had been in their rented property for less than a year, whereas this was true for only 8.2% of households in other tenures (Stone et al., 2013).[1] While the available data suggest that only around 20% of private tenant moves are forced moves, among some vulnerable groups the incidence of involuntary moves is far higher—42% for over 65s (Productivity Commission, 2019, p. 81).

Of course, many private renters who move house do so voluntarily for a range of reasons and may have little difficulty finding a new tenancy. However, as will be illustrated, in our study a proportion of renters, especially low-income earners, had great difficulty finding a property. In 1996, the Department of Social Security (DSS, 1996, p. 51) argued that the PRS (in Australia) was appropriate for "a dynamic and mobile society" as it provided "households with the capacity to relocate easily, and to respond to labour market and other exigencies without the commitment of capital …". The argument implies that all renters have equal capacity to move if they so desire and fails to recognise that such capability is structured by an individual's or household's resources. As Massey (1994, p. 156) referring to mobility argues,

> Different social groups have distinct relationships to this anyway-differentiated mobility: some are more in charge of it than others; some initiate flows and movement, others don't; some are more on the receiving end of it than others; some are effectively imprisoned by it.

Our research illustrates that a person's or household's ability to find a rental property is highly dependent on their financial capacity and other resources such as owning a vehicle and having internet at home. Low-income households are far more likely to struggle to find alternative accommodation and this battle can generate enormous anxiety. Noteworthy, is that our investigation found that even higher-income renters often had difficulty securing an alternative rental property that they felt met their needs.

A dwelling does not necessarily equate to a home: "A dwelling has become a home when its resident feels that it is the place in which he or she feels comfortable, secure, and relaxed" (Ruonavaara, 2012, p. 186). The sense that your dwelling is home is crucial "… as the environment where we spend a large proportion of our time – can have a significant impact on our identity and well-being" (Easthope, 2014, p. 581). Compared to social housing renters and home owners, the limited security and other

[1] This movement is accentuated by the large and highly mobile student renter population.

occupancy rights of private tenants in Australia restrict the potential for a rented dwelling to feel like home. PRS residents, more especially low-income households, have less power to control their situation (Hulse & Saugeres, 2008; Kemp, 2011; Morris, 2016). A tenant who perceives that there is an ever-present possibility that they will be asked to vacate or that their rent will be increased to an untenable level will, in all likelihood, find it difficult to feel at home (Desmond & Shollenberger, 2015). As Woodhall-Melnick et al. (2017, p. 255) conclude "… when individuals are unable to generate a narrative of housing stability in their narratives of the future, existential anxiety may result". The issue of insecurity and its impacts is examined in-depth in Chap. 7.

Whether an individual perceives their dwelling as home is shaped by a range of factors beyond their security of occupancy. As mentioned, privacy, physical condition, and scope for personalisation of the space are all important (Dupuis & Thorns, 1998; Easthope, 2004, 2014). The tenant's relationship with their landlord and/or real estate manager is critical. A landlord or property manager who disrespects their tenant, refuses to attend to legitimate concerns or enforces regulations perceived as unreasonable, will necessarily impact on a tenant's sense of home (Morris, 2016). As mentioned in Chap. 3, almost three quarters of tenants deal primarily with a real estate agent rather than their landlord, so the approach of the former can make a real difference to whether a tenant feels at home (Hulse et al., 2018). Beyond the dwelling, the neighbourhood can also be an important influence. In neighbourhoods that are unsafe, poorly located and or lacking in basic amenities, residents are less likely to feel at home (Kearns & Parkinson, 2001; Morris, 2019).

The home is a space where the resident should have the capacity to secure their privacy if they so desire (Karin-Frank, 2020; King, 2004). Tenants living in situations where their landlord or property manager feels they have the de facto right to impinge on their privacy, will find it difficult to create a sense of home. A major study of older private renters in the UK found that breaches of tenants' privacy by landlords were not unusual and that these breaches made them "feel on edge and was an invasion of their space …" (Fear et al., 2004).

Dwelling condition is another key variable likely to influence a resident's sense of home (Easthope, 2014; Fear et al., 2004). Although unsatisfactory housing conditions are certainly not confined to the PRS, it is probably more likely that private renters, more especially in low-rent areas, will experience poor maintenance and conditions[2] (Pawson & Herath, 2015; Productivity Commission, 2019).[3] Private renters rely on their landlord to maintain the property and not all landlords fulfil their obligations. This is especially so in the case of small investors who make up the majority of

[2]The cutbacks on expenditure on social housing has meant that maintenance has declined. The Productivity Commission's annual report on government services concluded that 20% of social housing dwellings in Australia do not meet minimum standards.

[3]In NSW residential tenancies legislation sets down seven minimum habitability standards—structural soundness, adequate lighting, ventilation, utilities, plumbing and drainage, water (including hot water), bathroom facilities, including toilet and washing and facilities with privacy. "Landlords need to ensure their rented properties meet the minimum standards to be fit for habitation" (NSW Government, 2020).

Australian landlords (Hulse et al., 2011). Further, private renters may be reluctant to ask landlords or agents to carry out maintenance works because they fear that the rent may be increased as a result or they may antagonise the landlord/real estate agent and jeopardise their tenancy (see Capstick et al., 2019). In our survey 18% of respondents said that they had decided "not to pursue or complain about a problem" because they feared that the landlord may ask them to leave or put up the rent.

The capacity for homemaking is important. If residents have "little say over the living space, it may not be easy to feel at home in it" (Ruonavaara, 2012, p. 186). A common restriction in the area of homemaking is a limitation on the renter's power to personalise the space; for example, tenants may not be allowed to knock nails in walls or do basic decorating like painting walls without obtaining the landlord's permission (Soaita & McKee, 2019).

Restrictions on the keeping of pets is not unusual and despite around two thirds of Australian households having a pet, a renter who has a companion animal may have severely restricted options (Power, 2017).[4] Not only are pet-friendly rental properties in short supply, but the ones that are available are often poor quality, making it difficult to create a sense of home (Power, 2017).

The remainder of the chapter examines how private renters go about finding a property and the challenges they may encounter. This is followed by an examination of how tenants view their ability to create a sense of home.

Finding a Rented Property

The backdrop to our Sydney and Melbourne research is the large and growing shortage of affordable rental housing in Australia's major cities. Thus in 2016 of the 384,000 very low income (bottom 20% of the national income distribution) private renting households, 80% nation-wide were subject to affordability stress—they were having to use more than 30% of their income to pay for their accommodation. In metropolitan areas, the comparable figure was 90% (Hulse et al., 2019). Most of the shortage was due to the non-availability of properties priced at no more than 30% of gross household income for this group.

For the quintile 2 (Q2) low-income households (households in receipt of income between the 20th and 40th percentile of the national distribution) there was a notional surplus of affordable rentals available to them nationally—although not necessarily in the right places. However, "the gross surplus for Q2 households becomes a national shortage of affordable and available rental housing when occupation by other income groups is taken into account" (Hulse et al., 2019, p. 36). The shortage of affordable rental accommodation, and the competition from middle and higher-income earners, puts low-income households in a difficult and vulnerable situation. It discourages them from leaving unsuitable housing (Morris, 2016; Soatia, 2020), and when

[4] Although under Victoria's 2020 rental reforms, a landlord must not unreasonably refuse a tenant's request to keep a pet.

moving is unavoidable, finding an alternative rental property is often difficult and can precipitate enormous anxiety.

The interviews demonstrated that the degree of difficulty tenants experienced finding a new and suitable rental property was dependent on a range of factors—financial resources were primary, however household composition, possessing pets, having a relationship with a landlord or real estate agent and where the person was prepared to live, were also key factors.

Gina (low-rent area, Sydney, married with two children) described her property search in a low-rent area in Sydney after a forced move. Her difficulty was related to her low income and having young children:

> Well, when you go [looking], like we found one house that we really liked in Rooty Hill [a low-income suburb in Sydney]. We got there and there was so many people. There were 30 applicants for the house. And the thing is like they were advertising it at say $480 a week, it was with so much interest people are willing to say, "Well I'll pay an extra $50 or $100" … and they're not allowed to do that, but they do it. And you know everyone else loses out, but I can't afford to offer that.

Families with school-age children are usually keen to stay in their present area. This compounded difficulties for Gina:

> There's at least more than 10 people every time we go to look at a property. We were looking at Penrith, but there's a new estate, Jordan Springs. They've got nice new homes, but then my kids don't want to leave their school and that's the thing. The kids, they don't want to change school. My daughter, she's in Year 10, she'll be going to Year 11 next year and I'm willing to make the travel but, … it's just, yeah, they want to stay in the area.

The last two properties Tracey (low-rent Sydney) had rented, had been sold forcing her to vacate. Finding a place for herself and three children was stressful:

> Yeah, a lot of stress and the rental market's horrible even out here in piddly old Mount Druitt.[5] There are 25 applicants per house. It's huge. The rental market is as fierce as hell and so naturally any landlord just picks the most attractive, highest income earner. What else would you pick … We actually stayed with mum for a spell.

The family landed up staying with Tracey's mother for an extended period as they waited for their future landlord to complete the renovation of the house next door to her mother. He had promised Tracey the house, but the renovation took much longer than anticipated.

For single parents finding a place can be especially challenging. Pam (low-rent Sydney) poignantly recounted her traumatic experience:

> Being left [by her partner] and you know having to find a house for me and five children was not easy … Like I would not have lived here, only that after like 35 applications [for a rented property] this one said, "Yes". Okay, I've got a house for my kids, let's go. So, like 35 applications. It was not an easy process. Especially you know, like for a single mum and having so many children too. They [real estate agents and landlords] were a bit wary I think … When you know like you are a single mum with five kids, they think like they're just going to run feral.

---

[5]Mount Druitt is about 45 km from the central business area and is one of Sydney's poorest suburbs.

Her difficulty was heightened by her having pets:

> I just didn't bother going to the ones that said, "No pets", and most of the time the houses were too small anyway cos I couldn't put a 17-year-old male in with a 12-year-old male. The boys need their own [space] and I couldn't put my 16-year-old daughter in with a two and four-year-old.

For older renters dependent on the Age Pension, finding a rental property in a housing market like Sydney or Melbourne is invariably intensely stressful. After Frank's partner died, his deceased partner's daughter gave him notice. He described how he felt:

> It was a shocking blow … You get the feeling of hopelessness because you've got nothing behind you. You're not a land owner and that's why it amazes me that people whinge about mortgages and all that. They don't really know what it's like.

Frank spent six months looking for affordable accommodation in Sydney but was not successful. Eventually he was forced to move to a village 300 km from Sydney where he had no social ties. He claimed that the stress of the search for an affordable rental dwelling ultimately led to him having a heart attack.

With affordable accommodation so difficult to find, Carol (67) felt she had little choice but to rent a property that was clearly unsuitable. It was far too small.

> It is very hard to get a place that's suitable for an older person especially if it is a female on her own … Safety [is an] issue, plus you know the housing not being available for older people. There's not enough villa type accommodation [she had mobility problems] at a reasonable rent ... I thought this might be one of the better areas and yeah, so I took the first one I looked at. Well others I looked at beforehand were very run down. Grotty, absolutely disgusting, so this was reasonably good you know, so I thought I better get here and hurry up.

Another interviewee dependent on the Age Pension, Bill (70) had a vehicle and was thus able to search across a wide area. Nevertheless, he almost found himself homeless:

> I'd had to move about five times in the last six years because people wanted to sell their house, so I got turfed out … and that put me at some stages in a very difficult position because you couldn't just go to an agent and rent something. You had to … compete for a premise [property] … The last rental was in Oberon and it took me seven weeks and 14 applications to find that … I applied in Penrith, Katoomba, Mudgee and Bathurst[6] and that's the only one I got … I was one day [away from being] out on my ear because the landlord waited three weeks before he made a decision … and that was one day before I had to move out of the other place …

Difficulty in finding rental accommodation is not confined to low-income households. Louise (high-rent area, Sydney) had a well-paid job:

> Looking is just ghastly you know … You go to look at a place that's halfway decent … and you know there's fifty other people there ... What the agents have started doing is when they know they're going to have a massive crowd or that they want to lease a place quickly, they offer it to view on a … weekday, so that cuts out a lot of people who can't come on that day. But I was able to get out of work and run down here in 10 minutes … and have a look and there was only me and another couple because the place was in such a bad state.

---

[6] Penrith is 124 km from Oberon. Bathurst is 145 km from Penrith.

Having a cat added to her struggle and accepting a place that she quickly realised was not suitable:

> The place was dark and damp, but the reason I jumped at it was because it was pet friendly. See this is another thing about renting. You can ... Yeah, you can rarely find places that accept pets and so I jumped at it for that reason.

Some interviewees had no difficulty finding an alternative rental property. Amivi (low-rent area, Melbourne) had lived in the same rental property for 20 years. After her husband died, she felt she had to move. Her excellent relationship with her real estate agent was crucial:

> I mentioned maybe [the real estate agent] could help me to find another place because I cannot stay there, because I have sad memories with my husband passing. So, they give me the rental list and... the first thing I saw was this one. I said, "Can I take it?" He said, "Okay, tomorrow 5 pm you can come." So, tomorrow 5 pm, I came. The [land]lady's here, so I came. When I go inside the kitchen, everything, I say, "I like this one".

Beth (high-rent area, Melbourne) said she had never had a problem finding alternative accommodation. The fact that she was single and in a high paying job, certainly helped:

> I've always found it easy to get somewhere to live at a price that I'm willing to pay. So I've never really had a problem.

Feeling at Home

Our Sydney/Melbourne renters survey suggested that most tenants felt at home in their rental property. About six in ten felt "very much at home", another 34% felt "somewhat at home" and only 5% said they did not feel at "home at all". Renters in low-rent areas were less likely to feel at home. Only 55% of these renters said that they felt very much at home, compared to 65% in medium and high-rent areas.

As outlined, the condition of the home, maintenance, the ability to personalise the space, the tenant's relationship with the landlord or real estate agent and finally the neighbourhood, are all key determinants of a private renter's capacity to create a sense of home. Although interrelated, they are discussed in turn.

Condition of the Dwelling

Although the condition of a person's residential property does not necessarily determine whether they feel at home, it can be a significant contributor (Easthope, 2014; Evans et al., 2000). Just over three quarters of our survey respondents said that their rental property is in good condition. The differences in the responses of renters in low, medium and high areas were not significant. However, there were significant differences ($p < 0.05$) between respondents ($n = 70$) reliant on government benefits (excluding people on the Age Pension) as compared with those receiving wages or salaries ($n = 443$). Whereas, 79% of the latter group agreed or strongly agreed that their dwelling was in good condition, only 63% of respondents on income support thought so. In response to the question, "To what extent do you agree or disagree with the statement … I am very satisfied with my home", only 6% of waged or salaried respondents disagreed or strongly disagreed with this statement. In strong contrast, this was true for one in four respondents reliant on government benefits.

The in-depth interviews provide more insight on these differences. They indicate that for a proportion of renters, especially government benefit reliant tenants in low-rent outer areas, the poor condition of their rented property made it difficult for them to feel at home. Sylvia, a single parent, lived in a run-down house with her five-year old son in the outer suburbs of Sydney. The kitchen floor had gritty linoleum that had not been replaced for many years, if ever. Heavy metal bars on the windows gave the house an oppressive feel. There was only an outside toilet. She described her initial impression:

> And as soon as I looked at the house I said, "Oh my god, a junkie house". It was full of cockroaches and the weeds were up to his [her five year-old's] window. Just crap everywhere. There's still broken glass and everything. If you go and pick up the stuff every day, you'd never get rid of it.

Despite its rundown state, she had to take it:

> I had no other option. It was either move here or live on the streets, I was stuck in a refuge, long story, but I had to take this place or I had nowhere else to live. I'm three years almost [here] … You know, nothing works properly. Handles break and stuff. Light fixtures have just shattered in the roof when I've tried to take light a globe out to change it. You know, shit like that.

Nigel's view was not dissimilar. He was unemployed and lived by himself in outer Sydney. His fibro home was in poor condition. There were curtains where there should have been doors, and the yard was chaotic. Nigel's assessment was definitive:

> This house here is a piece of shit. As you can see, it is just, it's not what you'd call up to standard.

The dire condition of the dwelling certainly had an impact on his ability to feel at home. When asked if he felt at home, he responded,

> Not at all. No, the only reason I'm stuck in the house is if I know someone's coming around … I hate being here. I only sleep here.

Carol (67) was frail and the Age Pension was her sole source of income. Her accommodation was far too small and on a steep hill which she struggled to negotiate. The small size and location made it extremely difficult for her to create a sense of home.

> All I could fit in was my bed and a lounge … I've got boxes and washing machine and dryer and everything sitting around the lounge room and the bedroom, so yeah there's not much room … It is very inadequate and it is too small. I'm finding it very difficult. Like four walls looking at you every day … I can't settle and it makes it really difficult to get interested and involved with anything because of where you live …

Fred and Winnie (low-rent area, Sydney) had more or less given up on resolving the various issues with their rental property. The drainage was so poor that when it rained it was difficult to venture out of the house. The house was damp and mould was a serious problem.[7] The landlord was evasive about resolving the various problems and had put the house on the market. The conditions made it difficult to create a sense of home:

> They [the landlords] don't seem to want to do too much and when it got too much, they decided to sell it. Sell it to some poor fool … They did put concrete down all around the house but because the lay of the land … all the water runs from the back … so when it's raining you can't go out unless you've got gum boots on … There's no drainage … Because of the dampness in the bedrooms, the clothes were going mouldy and I was noticing the other day when I was in our wardrobe, the ceiling in the wardrobe, the paint's peeled off.

Renters spoke of the unfortunate consequences of having to find a place in a rush. Louise (high-rent area, Sydney) was so unhappy with her apartment, that she broke her lease after only three weeks:

> Well there was massive traffic noise that I hadn't heard on the day that I went to look at it. And it [the traffic noise] was just so overwhelming that I couldn't live with it … So the whole thing became too much and after three weeks I just said, "You know, sod it. We (she and her thirteen-year-old daughter) can't live like this". Three weeks, it cost me just over $2,000 to get out of that lease, but I was prepared to pay it to get out of there and so we came here and thank goodness …

Louise had the financial resources to escape from her situation. Often, this is not the case.

Gina's home in outer Sydney was spotless, but it was cramped and old. The family felt sheepish about their accommodation and found it difficult to feel at home:

> We're comfortable, … but if we have the opportunity to go somewhere else, we will …. Even though it's all kept nice and clean, like other people in the family have got nicer homes and you just, I don't know, my partner gets a bit embarrassed and same as my daughter, but you know like our family know we've been living here in the neighbourhood. They know what the house is like. I don't know. You just feel a bit embarrassed sometimes.

Wells and Harris (2007) found that poor home quality can impact on how people view themselves. Gina's case appears to exemplify the way this can impact on self-esteem. It certainly had a profound impact on her 14 year-old daughter who "hated" the house:

> She hates this house; she absolutely hates it. She will not bring friends here and it's funny because one of her friends, her home is a lot worse than this, but she, I just don't know what it is, she just hates it.

Certainly, for a proportion of renters the condition of their home had an impact on their capacity to create a sense of home. However, the majority were satisfied with the condition of their rental property. Even in low-rent areas, many were living in

---

[7]Noteworthy is that a third of respondents to our survey agreed or strongly agreed that "mould or damp on ceiling, walls or floors [was] a problem".

adequate dwellings. Lynette loved her townhouse that she shared with her partner in outer Sydney and felt very much at home:

> Yes, I love it here and I love having my friends over and my family over … Three bedrooms, lots of storage, they've all got built-in wardrobes. There's also a walk in robe just off the main bedroom. It's got an on-suite. So luxurious I think is the word I'm looking for … So we've got our own bathrooms, we've got our own bedrooms. Two TV rooms if we want to watch something different we can … I've always wanted a townhouse …

How renters responded to the condition of their dwelling was also shaped by their general disposition and a trade-off against the rent paid. Stefan (low-rent, Sydney, no dependents) described his house where he had lived for 11 years as a "dump", but he was content. His contentment was premised on his easy-going disposition, a good relationship with his landlord, the suitability of the house for his job and importantly, the low rent.

> It's a dump. It is falling down … The whole place is bowed and sort of you know, it's basically a knock down so that gives me reasonably cheap rent because there's no money to be spent on the place … At the moment it works out rather well for me because I can basically do what I want. I can paint the whole place black if I wanted to. I get along really well with the landlord. I let him store timber and things for his concrete business here, so he's got to be nice to me, you know what I mean.

Although her apartment was a tiny studio, the bed folded into the wall, Myra was content and felt totally at home.

> Yeah, like I said to you, I hate things and I don't want anything and I work a lot. I'm addicted to my computer, so yeah. It actually suits me perfect.

Maintenance

When asked, "How satisfied are you with the landlord or agent's response when something needed to be fixed or repaired", about six in ten renters said that they were "satisfied" or "very satisfied", another 13% were neither satisfied or dissatisfied and one in five were dissatisfied or very dissatisfied. Interestingly, there were no significant differences between the high, medium and low-rent areas.

The response to maintenance requests is potentially highly significant for well-being and having a sense of home. Tenants who were in high end rental properties rarely had maintenance issues and when there was an issue they expected that the landlord respond, thus reinforcing other research finding that real estate agents found such tenants to have high expectations about timeliness of responses to requests (see Hulse et al., 2018). Amber lived in a luxurious home in one of the most expensive areas in Sydney. The home was in perfect condition and it was evident that the maintenance was exceptional:

> They [the landlord/ real estate agent] are very good. So we've got a gardener included. I said to them when we first looked at the place with all these hedges, I said, "There's no way I can manage those, can we include gardening on the lease?" And they did so, yeah. So the gardener comes, in winter it's every three weeks and in summer every two weeks … I mean you're in that sort of rent bracket, there are certain things like you've got to keep the place looking nice and tidy.

Yvonne (high-rent Sydney) had never had to contact her landlord:

> It's just like everything's fine. Everything works. Everything's in fairly good condition. So there's never been any dramas about anything like that. So no, I don't want to change anything. It's kind of perfect.

Not surprisingly, tenants who had landlords or agents who responded promptly and competently to maintenance requests, were more likely to feel at home in their accommodation. Prisha (low-rent area, Melbourne) was content in her accommodation and her excellent relationship with her landlord (rather than the agent), certainly contributed to her feeling at home in her rented property:

> Our owner is very nice, so whatever problem [we have] we just call. Suppose if we call the [real estate] agency and the agency takes some time and we … [happen to] see the owner … so we complain to him and he says, "Okay, I will take action".

The interviews suggested that in most instances landlords or agents were responsive to repairs that were absolutely necessary. Paul's (medium-rent area, Melbourne) assessment was typical:

> When the important stuff happens, like the oven breaks, they do fix that quickly so that's the important stuff, and that's good. When the air conditioner or heating broke they got in very quickly to fix it, so that's the main stuff.

Also, when the landlord is able to do the necessary repairs him/herself, it is more likely that they would be responsive and maintenance would be adequate. Patsy (low-rent, Melbourne) had a good relationship with her landlord and felt at home:

> I think the owner was fixing, the other day, fixing the window. And I think he's coming back, I'm not sure when. But he's going to fix the side of the roof. So every time we say something, he will come and fix it and he will give us a few days' notice and say, "I'm coming here".

In contrast, Michaela (low-rent outer Sydney) who had been in the same rental property for 16 years had given up on her landlord/estate agent responding to requests. The failure to respond, made it difficult for her to create a sense of home:

> Things I'd like to do, I can't do because I've requested for painting and things like that before on several occasions and it has never eventuated … Yeah, personally I would like to paint all through the house you know and tidy up and the do the outside exterior and everything, but what can you do. It is not yours. You can't do it … I want the house to, I want to be proud and be clean and you know appealing … and you can't do it you know. They say "No", so that's it. There's nothing you can do about it.

Like Michaela, Raelene (low-rent, Melbourne) felt disempowered. She lived in an apartment block and was struggling to get the body corporate (the owners)[8] to respond to her maintenance requests:

> When you are only renting and you are not an owner, and living in the house, it's very hard to get them to do anything … Myself and another couple of other neighbours have been persistently on their back to get things done. I mean it took about six years to get three huge trees cut down, which shouldn't be where they were.

A number of tenants mentioned the reluctance of their landlords/estate agents to commit to maintenance that was not absolutely essential and perhaps costly to undertake:

> Every year they come out and every year I say exactly the same thing to them, and I complain about exactly the same issues that I've got – big cracks and things like that. Each year it's the same. They wander away [saying], "You're doing a good job with the property," and I don't really see them again. But I have to credit them in that when something big goes wrong, it doesn't take them long to come. (Lenka, low-rent, Melbourne)

Graham (high-rent area, Sydney) had a similar problem to Lenka. Asked about the landlord's attitude to maintenance, he responded:

> Yeah, they're sort of okay. We've asked them to do certain things and they haven't bothered because they're too expensive [to repair] which is fair enough, so we put up with that and the rent is sort of, it's a reasonable rent, so we don't sort of make unreasonable demands … They're quite good with maintenance. Things like plumbing, electricity and stuff like that.

As discussed, in a tight rental market like Sydney or Melbourne, finding affordable rental accommodation is difficult especially for low-income households. Tenants were determined to hang on to their accommodation even if it meant having to endure poor maintenance. Pam was typical of tenants who decided it was better to avoid being too demanding:

> When I complained about the last rental increase, they [the agent] said, "Write down everything that's wrong and refuse to pay it until everything is fixed …". I was like, I'm just lucky to have somewhere to live. I'm not going to bother about it … When you're a single parent on a pension … No, at the time it was like just shut up and cop it sweet. I'm not going to rock the boat. I'm not on a lease anymore. Let it go. If that's what he [the landlord] feels he needs to do, let him do it.

Julie (medium-rent, Sydney) had little storage space. She was reluctant to request that the landlord install more:

> I don't want the rent to go up. I mean I'd pay a bit more if that could be negotiated, but I don't want to be seen as a difficult tenant, I think that's really what it is. Like once you start asking for stuff, "Oh no, there's that annoying tenant that's asking for this". I feel like you just get put into a category … I'm trying not to rock the boat. I really think that's what it is. I just keep my head down.

---

[8]The body corporate governs apartment blocks and makes decisions about maintenance of the exterior and common areas. It is constituted only by owners. Renters are not represented.

Gina had no compunction about reporting problems, but was concerned that making too much fuss would be weaken her relationship with the landlord and would be held against her the next time she needed to find rented accommodation:

> I don't feel restrained asking them, but I mean if they weren't to go ahead [with repairs], if they were flat out to say "No", well really, what do you do? You either cop it and go, "Yeah fine, he's not going to do it", or you take the chance of making a formal complaint through the correct people,[9] but then I feel that that goes against you ... Yeah, and I just don't see why you could have to wait months for your hearing to come up and ... I think it just makes the relationship with you know yourself and the real estate and the landlord a bit more shaky which is wrong cos it is there to help you, but in the end I don't think it does, so it's catch 22.

The Relationship of the Tenant with the Landlord/Estate Agent and Feeling at Home

The relationship tenants have with their landlord and or estate agent can be a central determinant of whether a tenant feels at home. Clark and Kearns (2012, p. 934) conclude,

> Landlords' overall service performance, how they keep tenants informed and how they take tenants' views on board, all make a difference to ratings of home quality and to psychosocial status and control.

Tenants who felt that they were treated respectfully were more liable to feel at home and to help maintain the property. Also, when tenants had a direct and good relationship with the landlord, there appeared to be more capacity for tenants to personalise their abode. Leon, married with two children, lived in a four-bedroomed house next door to his landlords (a couple). His relationship with his landlords was exceptional. He had a particularly high regard for them.

> They're very kind and generous people and they're not the sort of person that would get this as a property investment and try and make money on it and turn it over every six months.

His excellent relationship meant that he was prepared to do a good deal of maintenance:

> Well, I do all the yards and front lawn ... I get her [the landlord] over and we go gardening together. So we do all that ... The roof fell in, so I fixed the roofs ... I do all the maintenance on the inside.

The capacity of tenants to makes changes and personalise their living space certainly contributed towards renters feeling at home. The interviews indicated that Lenka's (low rent, Melbourne) landlord was very obliging:

---

[9]Gina is referring to the NSW Civil & Administrative Tribunal that endeavours to resolve tenants' disputes with landlords.

> The one thing that I was really grateful with him was he's basically said, "Treat it as your home … You can do what you like to the garden". He said, "So far as things like interior painting and stuff like that, don't make it garish". He's given me a guideline as to what I can and can't do.

Like Lenka, Prisha (low-rent Melbourne) was able to personalise the space:

> If we want to buy any decoration or anything, we just buy it. We don't think that this is not our home. We just buy it and make it [the way we want] ... Yeah, we don't feel that it is not our home … We don't feel like that because after all we are living here the last ten years, so it is our home.

Similarly, Tracey's landlord was easy-going and allowed her to make major changes:

> We have a really approachable landlord who will let me repaint or, at the moment I'm about to speak to him about pulling up one of the bedroom's carpet and he can see his stylish floor that he put in. I'm going to paint the floorboards in that bedroom as well, rather than have the carpet.

Sonia (Sydney, medium-rent) had a similar relationship with her landlord:

> Yeah, we feel very much at home. Sometimes it's hard to believe that it is not ours and you know it'd be hard to explain to our five-year-old why this house is not ours …

More affluent tenants had the capacity to be innovative in regards to personalising the space and not causing damage. Brooke (high-rent, Sydney) felt that the capacity to personalise the space was essential and had set up a sophisticated system to hang up her "pictures":

> Yeah, because look the first thing that will make you feel homey and cosy is books, cushions, pictures. Look, I've lived in a lot of apartments and I know that they're the things that you need. If a wall is blank it doesn't have much feeling or invitingness to it. So basically, the whole hall is pictures. And look I've had to pay extra to get a proper system to be able to do that, so it's a gallery system. So it is one wire, but you can hang multiple frames on it … As soon as you walk in, you feel warm and invited.

Some tenants who were handy and felt at home, appeared to spend a good deal of time and sometimes money personalising their accommodation. Tomas (medium rent, Sydney) was highly involved in maintaining his rented property:

> He [the landlord] knows that you know, I'm not thrashing the place … If anything, I've just added maybe $20,000 to $30,000 value to it just on simple little repairs and fixing up bits and pieces around the place. Yeah, I don't think there's been a single weekend where I haven't been … fixing something here and there.

Philip (medium-rent, Melbourne) had a strong sense of home and had embarked on various modifications to personalise his rented property:

> It's all fine. I tinker with things when I need to. I put speakers out in the garage for music and … I just put in some fluorescent lights in the garage to play games out there, and I just do that … I just tend to hang things where I want to hang them. I don't ask them. I just do it.

In contrast, Graham (high-rent area, Sydney) was capable of doing major repairs, but was frustrated by the restrictions placed on him and believed they had an impact on his family's capacity to create a sense of home.

> Well it is frustrating not being able to do things. Like there's various things when you're living in a place you'd like to do. Simple things like putting up pictures on the walls - there's restrictions on those. And I mean we'd like a window in the bedroom to let the sun in, but obviously we can't do that … We don't make suggestions that we think are going to scare the owners … You never really feel like it's your home. It is always in the back of your mind that you can't do things with it that you'd like to do.

When tenants are prepared to pay for items, landlords are far more amenable. The semi-detached home, Graham and family were living in, was extremely cold in winter. They decided to install a gas connection for their heater:

> They didn't have this heater outlet here when we came, so we said, "Well we don't want to freeze during winter", so we actually paid to put that in and they were happy with that, obviously so.

Not surprisingly, research has indicated that interventions that improve heating in a home do impact on the happiness and wellbeing of the occupants (Howden-Chapman et al., 2007).

Renters with disposable income who saw their rental property as home in the long-term, were prepared to spend money to make their home more comfortable. Sarah had grown up in a rented property and had a different mind-set to her husband:

> And when I want to make improvements he [her husband] thinks, "Let's not invest money in somebody else's property." And I have a different mindset and say, "We're investing in our home. We're living here. It might be their property, but this is our home, so I want to make it comfortable for me because this is my life".

Gina (low-rent area, Sydney) was frustrated by her inability to decorate. Asked what the drawbacks of long-term renting are, she responded, "And just not being able to do, even though it's your home you're living there you know if there's things that you want to do, you've always got to get permission to do things". She was also concerned about spending money on a rented property:

> My daughter would like to paint [her room]. Like I'm sure that they'd give us permission, but we just, you do get worried about putting money in when you don't know really how long you've got [in the property]. Like we could go and paint and make it all look much better, but you know, are you going to do that at every house that you go to?

Pets can be a major issue. Besides restricting the choices renters have (see Power, 2017), they can antagonize landlords. Graham felt that there was a link between a recent rent increase and the family having a large dog:

> We unfortunately had the owners come around at the last inspection and they hadn't been here for about three years I suppose and they complained about the dog … We were very specific that we had the dog on the lease, but they said the house smelled of dogs, so they weren't too impressed with that and they decided to put up the rent and whether they wanted us to move we're not quite sure, but we balanced that and said, "No, it was cheaper for us to stay here and we want to stay", so we copped the extra rent increase.

Personalising the home was made difficult in certain instances by landlords not respecting the private space of tenants. Tomas's landlord was especially meddling and not consultative:

> So on several occasions actually I got phone calls saying I'm coming over this afternoon which I find a bit intrusive. One occasion he brought his brother over and they were talking about renovating the kitchen, bathroom and laundry and basically said for three weeks there just won't be a kitchen, bathroom and laundry.

The Neighbourhood

Perceptions of the neighbourhood has been shown to be an important influence in shaping whether residents feel at home. Clark and Kearns (2012, p. 934) conclude:

> How residents feel about their neighbourhood, and how they perceive others to view their neighbourhood are related to both their perceptions of home quality, and their feelings of status and control.

Certainly, many of our research participants felt at home, not only because they were satisfied with their own accommodation, but also because they had a strong affinity with the neighbourhood. Convenience was a key factor: "Yeah, I like it because it's close by for me, for everything. I take my trolley and go when I have to do a little shopping" (Ingrid, low-rent area, Melbourne).

The ability to walk to work and amenities was a big factor. Anne and her partner lived in a high-rent area in inner Melbourne:

> We love living here. There's lots of nice places to eat and we can walk to the Vic Market and do our shopping. And I can walk into the city which is convenient and it's really easy commuting because my work changes because I'm a freelancer … The train station is a hub, and so it's got trains every few minutes, and we've got a tram line, and Peter (partner) can walk to work or he can ride.

Social ties in the area were also important. Prisha had a good deal of contact with her fellow tenants and felt she could definitely call on them if necessary. That her neighbours were all originally from India was a factor:

> Our three neighbours which are all from our mother country … so that's why we have a good relationship with them and one neighbour is here. We have a good relationship with him also.

Amber's social circle appeared to be concentrated in her neighbourhood:

> Another reason I don't want to leave Mosman [Sydney] is we've got a lot of really good friends that have been very supportive. You know when you have the tough times it is nice and you've got people that will help you out …

A few interviewees were deeply unhappy with their neighbourhood and did not feel at home as a result. When asked if she would stay local if they moved, Winnie (low-rent, Sydney) responded,

> We'd like to get out of it. It is getting worse. We had a drive-by shooting a couple of streets behind us last week. Where we are here it's great, but you drive around the corner and … it is pretty unsavoury. I won't go out at night ... Once darkness comes, that's it. Lock all the doors. You don't feel really safe in your own house either.

Conclusions

The psychosocial environment in which a person resides is viewed as a key determinant of wellbeing and feeling at home is a central component thereof (see Clarke & Kearns, 2012; Easthope, 2014). The data indicate that most renters are able to create a sense of home. The quality of the rental property, their relationship with the landlord/real estate agent, general maintenance, the perceived quality of the neighbourhood and security of tenure, are all contributory factors. Certainly, tenants' relationship with the landlord and/or the agent is foundational. Tenants who are not harassed, can personalise the space, feel they can make requests without fear and that the requests will be responded to, are more likely to feel a sense of home.

The capacity to create a sense of home certainly does vary. It is partially a function of contingency; some tenants are unfortunate and find themselves in situations where it is difficult to feel at home, perhaps due to unexpected issues like traffic noise, unpleasant neighbours, an intrusive landlord or real estate agent or a sense that they can be asked to vacate at any time. Alternatively, they may be fortunate and find themselves in accommodation which is owned by a congenial and helpful landlord/real estate agent who endeavour to respond to all reasonable requests.

However, the primary source of variation is the varying financial capacity of tenants. Although not all of our interviewees in high and medium-rent areas reported a strong sense of home, our evidence indicates that tenants in low-rent areas are more likely to be in situations where the condition of their accommodation, maintenance and the landlord's responsiveness to requests is unsatisfactory. This was especially so among renters in low-rent areas in Sydney. This is not surprising. In an expensive rental market, the choices of low-income individuals/households are limited. This is particularly so for those reliant on welfare benefits. Often they are forced to accept unsuitable accommodation and to reside in non-preferred neighbourhoods. Their capacity to feel at home in these circumstances is necessarily limited. Also, their accommodation is more likely to be controlled by a landlord or real estate agent who does not facilitate the creation of a sense of home. There is a realisation by the landlord/agent that the power of a low-income tenant to press their demands is limited. They do not have the financial resources to relocate easily. Also, tenants are well-aware that landlords can ask them to vacate without the need to provide reasons (no grounds eviction). Landlords and agents are generally more responsive to higher income tenants as there is a realisation that these tenants have the capacity to find alternative accommodation and a vacancy can cost the landlord and agent a significant amount. It also perhaps a cultural capital issue. Higher income tenants are more likely to know what their rights are as tenants (see Hulse et al., 2018).

References

Capstick, N., Gardiner, J., Murray, J., Mowbray, J., & Patterson Ross, L. (2019). *Lives turned upside down: NSW renters' experience of 'no grounds' eviction*. Sydney: Tenants' Union of NSW & Marrickville Legal Centre.

Clark, J., & Kearns, A. (2012). Housing improvement, perceived housing quality and psychological benefits from the home. *Housing Studies, 27*(7), 915–939.

Desmond, M., & Shollenberger, T. (2015). Forced displacement from rental housing: Prevalence and neighbourhood consequences. *Demography, 52*(5), 1751–1771.

Department of Social Security. (1996). *Overview of the Australian private rental market*. Canberra: Australian Government.

Dufty-Jones, R. (2012). Moving home: Theorizing housing within a politics of mobility. *Housing, Theory and Society, 29*(2), 207–222.

Dupuis, A., & Thorns, D. (1998). Home, home ownership and the search for ontological security. *Sociological Review, 46*(1), 24–47.

Easthope, H. (2004). A place called home. *Housing, Theory and Society, 21*(3), 128–138.

Easthope, H. (2014). Making a rental property home. *Housing Studies, 29*(5), 579–595.

Evans, G., Wells, N. M., Chan, H. E., & Saltsman, H. (2000). Housing quality and mental health. *Journal of Consulting and Clinical Psychology, 68*(3), 526–530.

Fear, T., Carlton, N., Heywood, F., Izuhara, M., Pannell, J., & Means, R. (2004). Home or hell: Older tenants' experiences in the private rented sector. *The Journal of Adult Protection, 6*(2), 15–20.

Heylen, K., & Van den Broeck, K. (2016). Discrimination and selection in the Belgian private rental market. *Housing Studies, 31*(2), 223–236.

Howden-Chapman, P., Matheson, A., Crane, J., Viggers, H., Cunningham, M., Blakely, T., Cunningham, C., Woodward, A., Saville-Smith, K., O'Dea, D., Baker, M., Waipara, N., Chapman, R., & Davie, G. (2007). Effect of insulating existing houses on health inequality: Cluster randomised study in the community. *BMJ, 334*, 460–464.

Hulse, K., & Saugeres, L. (2008). *Housing insecurity and precarious living in Australian rental housing*, No. 124. Melbourne: Australian Housing and Urban Research Institute (AHURI).

Hulse, K., Reynolds, M., Nygaard, C., & Yates, J. (2019). *The supply of affordable private rental housing in Australian cities: Short-term and longer-term changes*. Melbourne: AHURI (Australian Housing and Urban Research Institute).

Hulse, K., Martin, C., James, A., & Stone, W. (2018). *Private rental in transition: Institutional change, technology and innovation in Australia,* No. 296. Melbourne: AHURI (Australian Housing and Urban Research Institute).

Hulse, K., Milligan, V., & Easthope, H. (2011). *Secure occupancy in rental housing: Conceptual foundations and comparative perspectives,* No. 170. Melbourne: AHURI (Australian Housing and Urban Research Institute).

Karin-Frank, S. (2020). Homelessness, the right to privacy, and the obligation to provide a home. In G. J. M. Abbarno (Ed.), *The ethics of homelessness: Philosophical perspectives*. Leiden: Koninklijke Brill NV.

Kearns, A., & Parkinson, M. (2001). The significance of neighbourhood. *Urban Studies, 38*(12), 2103–2110.

Kemp, P. A. (2011). Low-income tenants in the private rental sector. *Housing Studies, 26*(7), 1019–1034.

King, P. (2004). *Private dwelling: Contemplating the use of housing*. London: Routledge.

MacDonald, H., Nelson, J., Galster, G., Paradies, Y., Dunn, K., & Dufty-Jones, R. (2016). Rental discrimination in the multi-ethnic metropolis: Evidence from Sydney. *Urban Policy and Research, 34*(4), 373–385.

Massey, D. (1994). *Space, place and gender*. Cambridge: Polity Press.

Morris, A. (2016). *The Australian Dream: Housing experiences of older Australians*. Melbourne: CSIRO Publishing.

Morris, A. (2019). *Gentrification and displacement: The forced relocation of public housing tenants in Inner-Sydney*. Singapore: Springer.

NSW Government. (2020). *Changes to the residential tenancy laws*. Sydney: NSW Fair Trading, NSW Government.

Pawson, H., & Herath, S. (2015). *Disadvantaged places in urban Australia: Residential mobility, place attachment and social exclusion*, No. 243. Melbourne: AHURI (Australian Housing and Urban Research Institute).

Power, E. R. (2017). Renting with pets: A pathway to housing insecurity? *Housing Studies, 32*(3), 336–360.

Productivity Commission, P. (2018). *Report on government services*. Canberra: Australian Government, Productivity Commission.

Productivity Commission, P. (2019). *Vulnerable private renters: Evidence and options*. Canberra: Australian Government, Productivity Commission.

Ruonavaara, H. (2012). Tenure as an institution. In S. Smith (Ed.), *International encyclopaedia of housing and home*. Amsterdam: Elsevier.

Soaita, A. M., & McKee, K. (2019). Assembling a 'kind of' home in the UK private renting sector. *Geoforum, 103*, 148–157.

Soatia, A., Munro, M., & McKee, K. (2020). *Private renters' housing experiences in lightly regulated markets*. Glasgow: UK Collaborative Centre for Housing Evidence. https://housingevidence.ac.uk/wp-content/uploads/2020/04/200429_PRS_evidence_review_final.pdf.

Stone, W., Burke, T., & Hulse, K. (2013). *Long-term private rental in a changing Australian private rental sector*. Melbourne: AHURI (Australian Housing and Urban Research Institute). https://www.ahuri.edu.au/__data/assets/pdf_file/0013/2227/AHURI_Final_Report_No209_Long-term-private-rental-in-a-changing-Australian-private-rental-sector.pdf.

Victorian Equal Opportunity and Human Rights Commission. (2012). *Locked out: Discrimination in Victoria's private rental market*. Carlton: Victorian Equal Opportunity and Human Rights Commission.

Wells, N. M., & Harris, J. D. (2007). Housing quality, psychological distress, and the mediating role of social withdrawal: A longitudinal study of low-income women. *Journal of Environmental Psychology, 27*(1), 69–87.

Woodhall-Melnik, J., Hamilton-Wright, S., Daoud, N., Matheson, F. I., Dunn, J. R., & O'Campo, P. (2017). Establishing stability: Exploring the meaning of 'home' for women who have experienced intimate partner violence. *Journal of Housing and the Built Environment, 32*, 253–268.

Chapter 6
Private Renting and Rental Stress

Abstract This chapter examines housing affordability in the PRS. We first discuss the concept of rental stress and its prevalence in Australia. The literature on housing affordability and wellbeing is then briefly reviewed. Drawing on our 2015 renters' survey in Sydney and Melbourne, the financial hardship faced by tenants in different housing markets is assessed. What is evident is that renters in low-rent areas are far more likely to be reliant on government benefits for their income, have an unemployed household member and have three or more financial stress indicators. The interviews we conducted are then utilised to examine rental stress for tenants reliant on government benefits. It was apparent that most were battling to cope with everyday expenses and that the resultant stress was often severe. Older private renters dependent on the Age Pension, the next group focused on, were in similar circumstances. Their rent consumed a considerable proportion of their income and this was having a deleterious impact on their capacity to lead a decent life. We then focused on tenants who were employed. In some households where only one member was employed rental stress was still evident. However, rental stress was not evident for households with two members employed.

Introduction

A key concern in Australia is the extent to which rents are affordable to households of different types, different income levels and those renting in different types of housing markets (Hulse et al., 2019; Productivity Commission, 2019). This chapter first defines and discusses the concept of rental stress and then briefly reviews the literature on housing affordability and wellbeing. Drawing on our 2015 renters' survey in Sydney and Melbourne, we then look at why rental stress matters and the financial hardship faced by tenants in different housing markets. This is followed by a discussion of the impact of rental stress on three groups—renters mainly or solely reliant on government benefits for their income; renters reliant on the government Age Pension[1] and lastly, renter households with employed members.

[1] Although the Age Pension is also a government benefit, we decided to treat people on the Age Pension as a separate category as older renters often have specific challenges.

A. Morris et al., *The Private Rental Sector in Australia*,
https://doi.org/10.1007/978-981-33-6672-5_6

Rental Stress: Defining the Problem

The concept of rental stress is premised on the understanding that affordable housing is a fundamental precondition for wellbeing. Rental housing that is expensive in relation to a household's income can leave the person, couple or family/household with insufficient funds to meet the cost of other essentials such as food or energy costs. There are two primary ways of measuring rental stress—the "ratio approach" and the "residual income" approach (AHURI, 2019; Burke et al., 2011; Stone, 2006; Yates & Gabriel, 2006). In Australia, the ratio approach (which is the preferred approach) is often called the "30:40 rule". A household is viewed as having a housing affordability problem or being in "rental stress" if they are on a low-income (defined as households in the bottom 40% of Australia's income distribution) and having to devote more than 30% of their income to pay for accommodation. Rental stress is confined to low-income households on the basis that better off groups will usually be able to afford to spend more than 30% of household income on housing without it affecting their expenditure on essential items (Nepal et al., 2010; Pawson et al., 2020; Rowley & Ong, 2012). As Pawson et al. (2020, p. 59) conclude,

> Implicitly the 30:40 rule assumes that households paying more than 30% of their housing in the top three quintiles of the income distribution are choosing to do so because they can afford it.

The second main way of measuring rental stress is the "residual income" method (Burke et al., 2011; Pawson et al., 2020; Stone, 2006). It is based on "budget standards" for households of different types/sizes and how much money is required to meet a minimum or modest standard of living through expenditure on non-housing items (see Saunders & Bedford, 2018). If there is insufficient income to pay rent after meeting one of these standards, the household has a housing affordability problem and is in rental stress (Burke et al., 2011). The residual income method enables greater nuance as it takes into account household type and size, but is more complex in terms of data for measurement and requires agreement on budget standards (Padley & Marshall, 2019).

It is important to recognise that households may move into and out of rental stress as their circumstances change (Baker et al., 2015; Rowley et al., 2015). Those who experience rental stress for an extended period are particularly vulnerable as over time they may have to forego more and more essential items. Rowley and Ong (2012) found that health and wellbeing declined substantially when households were in housing stress for three years or more.

There is a subjective element to rental stress. Households that appear to be in the same situation may perceive their situation differently. Thus Rowley and Ong (2012, p. 9) found,

> … there are households that fall within the traditional measure of stress that consider their levels of wellbeing acceptable. Additionally, there are households that fall outside the measure that are suffering considerable economic and social hardships.

Despite the limitations of the ratio definition and a recognition that there will certainly be exceptions, the research suggests that the 30:40 rule is useful as a broad-brush measure of rental stress and that this type of stress, particularly if experienced over the long term, may affect the health and wellbeing of these renters. What is far less contentious is that almost all private renter households who are in the bottom 20% (Q1) of the Australian household income distribution will be in rental stress and there will likely be consequences for wellbeing due to an inability to purchase essential items and anxiety about their future housing security (see Robinson & Adams, 2008).This will include households who are reliant on government benefits for their income, a major focus of this Chapter. Drawing on census data, Hulse et al. (2019) estimated that in 2016, 80% of Q1 private renter households were in rental stress.

The 2019 federal government (Productivity Commission) report on "vulnerable private renters" (defined as those on low income, bottom 40%) concluded that, by 2017–2018, two thirds of this group were spending more than 30% of their income on rent. The number of affected households doubled between 1994–1995 and 2017–2018 to reach about 710,000 (Productivity Commission, 2019).[2] A startling finding is that of the approximately one million low-income households in the PRS (about 2.65 million people) in 2017–2018, just under half had less than $500 a week remaining after paying the rent and 18% (170,000 households) had less than $250 (Productivity Commission, 2019).[3] In contrast, only 3% of other renting households had less than $500 a week.

Noteworthy is that the capacity of low-income households to escape rental stress appears to have diminished over the last two decades. In 2001, only a third of low-income tenants remained in rental stress four years on, whereas in 2016 about half of these households were still in rental stress four years later (Productivity Commission, 2019, p. 9). This finding is an important counter to the argument that rental stress is often only a temporary situation and therefore of minimal concern (Baker et al., 2015). A major concern going forward is that whereas historically a large proportion of private renters were able to escape rental stress by ultimately accessing employment or a better paid job, the Covid-19 pandemic and the consequent economic contraction will, in all likelihood, result in many more households in the PRS finding themselves in rental stress for extended periods or even life-long, as we discuss further in Chapter 8.[4]

Australian governments have recognised that low-income private renters experience rental stress. Many of those on pensions/benefits and family payments receive an additional payment called Rent Assistance (RA, see Chapter 1 for a discussion of RA) to offset some of the additional costs of renting. While any extra money is helpful in alleviating rental stress, the impact of the payment has gradually weakened due to maximum payment rates not keeping up with rent increases over the last two decades (Productivity Commission, 2019, p. 114). In 2018, 68% of households

---

[2]In 2016 there were 9,204,600 households in Australia (ABS, 2019).

[3]The poverty line in March 2018 other than housing was $507.43 per week for couples and $349 for sole person households (Melbourne Institute, 2018).

[4]In April 2020, employment fell by almost 600,000 after the lockdown imposed by the federal and state governments in response to Covid-19 (ABS, 2020).

receiving RA (over 1.3 million households) would have been in rental stress if they had not received it, but that number remains at 40% even when RA receipt is taken into account. This is despite about 80% of government benefit beneficiaries receiving the maximum RA amount in 2018, up from 57% in 2001 (Productivity Commission, 2019). Noteworthy, is that not all low income PRS households are eligible for the payment with working singles and couples without children on low wages missing out.

Rental Stress is About Rents Relative to Household Incomes

Rental stress is the result of the intersection between household incomes and rent levels. Looking firstly at rents, a big part of the problem is a dwindling supply of private rental dwellings which are affordable for low-income households using the 30% benchmark. Hulse et al. (2019), drawing on the 2016 ABS Census data, determined that nation-wide for Q1 (bottom 20% of income) households there was a shortage of 212,000 affordable dwellings and that the shortage increased to 305,000 due to many affordable dwellings being occupied by renters with higher incomes. Alarmingly, nationally 80% of Q1 private renter households were paying unaffordable rents and in metropolitan areas, 89% were (92% in Sydney). In 2016, for a Q1 household to avoid being in rental stress, they needed to find a dwelling with a rent at or below $202 per week. This was virtually impossible in Sydney and Melbourne. In Sydney the median rent at this time was around $500 a week and in Melbourne, $400.

Although there was a theoretical surplus of 491,000 private rental dwellings for Q2 households, many of these dwellings were occupied by middle and high-income earners. This resulted in a national shortage of 173,000 affordable and available dwellings for Q2 households. Close to half (46%) of Q2 households in the metropolitan areas were in rental stress (Hulse et al., 2019), indicating that rental stress has been moving higher up the household income scale particularly in large capital cities.

The other side of the rental stress problem is increasingly uncertain household incomes. Changes in the labour market such as an increase in casual and contract work, unemployment, underemployment and zero hours contracts have made household income increasingly difficult to predict (Whelan & Parkinson, 2017; Campbell et al., 2014). Within this labour market context, changes in income can also be precipitated by other types of disruptive life events such as relationship breakdown, domestic violence, and mental and physical health problems.

Although the growth of the PRS over the last two decades has been driven by all income groups, as discussed in Chapter 1, growth has been especially strong among low-income households. Within this group, private renter households reliant on government benefits for their income, are particularly vulnerable. The 2020 annual survey of rental affordability by Anglicare (an NGO linked to the Anglican church) applying an affordability test based on 30% of household income demonstrated the inadequacy of government pension/benefit rates in relation to prevailing rents. For example, just 526 (0.8%) of the 69,960 properties listed for rent across Australia on the 21 March 2020 were affordable for a single person on the Age Pension. Only 1.5% of advertised properties were affordable to "JobSeeker"[5] payment recipients, even factoring in the temporary increase to the payment enacted in March 2020 in response to the COVID-19 pandemic (Anglicare, 2020).

Another annual survey of rents, the Rental Affordability Index concluded that in 2019, using the median rent as a benchmark, that in Sydney a single person reliant on Newstart (the name of the unemployment benefit at that time) would have to use 135% of their income for rent (106% in Melbourne) and a single person on the Age Pension 88% (in Melbourne 67%) (SGS Economics & Planning, 2019).

Importantly, research shows that there is a spatial dimension in response to rental stress. Within the metropolitan cities such as Sydney and Melbourne, the more affordable dwellings are overwhelmingly in the outer suburbs which are often remote from jobs and long commuting times are thus a significant burden for many low-income households (see SGS Economics & Planning, 2019; Yates & Milligan, 2007). Many of these areas have poor public transport, so low-income households are dependent on private vehicles which can be costly to run (Rosier & McDonald, 2011).

The Impact of Rental Stress on Wellbeing

Although it is difficult to attribute causality, the available evidence suggests that rental stress can have serious implications more broadly for individual and household wellbeing (Morris, 2018; Robinson & Adams, 2008; Sweet et al., 2013). A study by Bentley et al. (2016, p. 216) drawing on HILDA data showed that "private renters whose housing became unaffordable experienced a small but significant decline in mental health". A more recent analysis of the HILDA data found "housing affordability to be a substantial potential driver of people's poor mental especially people who have low mental health to start with" (Baker et al., 2020, p. 5). Yates and Milligan (2007) concluded that a shortage of money to pay the rent and the resultant stress contributed to health problems and put stress on relationships. Also drawing on the HILDA data, Mallett et al. (2011) found that people living in unaffordable housing were more likely to report the worst mental health.

> Compared to those reporting the best (top 20%) mental health across the previous three years, those reporting the worst (bottom 20%) mental health were almost twice as likely to be in unaffordable housing. (Mallett et al., 2011, p. 6)

Outside of Australia, there is also evidence of rental stress affecting psychological wellbeing. Taylor et al. (2007) used data from waves 1 to 13 of the BHPS (British Household Panel Survey) to examine the impacts of housing payment problems on the

---

[5]In March 2020, the government changed the name of the unemployment benefit from Newstart to JobSeeker. At the same time the benefit was doubled to $1100 a fortnight. The doubling of the benefit is supposed to end in September 2020.

psychological wellbeing of renters and homeowners. They concluded that "raw data indicate strong relationships between unsustainable housing commitments, negative financial events and psychological wellbeing" (Taylor et al., 2007, p. 1031).

A US study compared 1419 respondents reporting high levels of stress regarding paying their rent or mortgage, to 1610 who indicated moderate stress and 6251 who reported low levels of stress (Herrick & Bona, 2013). The study concluded that "respondents in the high stress group, compared to the low stress group, had statistically significantly higher model-adjusted rates for all eight of the health-related outcomes examined" (p. 5) and that the results "demonstrate that housing stress is an independent risk factor associated with poor health outcomes, including diabetes, depression, hypertension and reduced access to medical care" (p. 5).

An analysis of the Housing Vacancy Survey, a representative survey conducted by the US Census bureau of more than 16,000 households in New York City, concluded "that housing cost burden is a risk factor for poor health and the postponement of health care services … [and] that the results suggest that housing cost burden exerts a stronger effect on health than certain measures of physical adequacy" (Metzler & Schwartz, 2016, p. 101). Not surprisingly, the greater the housing cost burden, the greater the impact on health.

Financial Hardship in Low Versus Medium/High Rent Areas in Sydney and Melbourne

Our survey of private tenants in low (outer suburban), medium (middle suburb) and high-rent (inner suburb) areas in Sydney and Melbourne indicated that rental stress has a significant spatial component. Not surprisingly, as indicated in Table 6.1, tenants in these different rental markets had very different profiles with respect to sources of income and employment status. Thus a third of households in low-rent

Table 6.1 Sources of income, employment status and recipients of Commonwealth rent Assistance by rental area

	Rent areas	
	Low ($n = 200$)	High and medium ($n = 399$)
	%	%
Wage or salaries as main source of household income	56	83
State pensions or benefits (including Age Pension) as main source of household income	33	7
Households having at least one member who was unemployed and seeking work	28	8
Rent Assistance recipients	62	21

Source Authors' survey 2015

areas were reliant primarily on government benefits for their income compared to 7% in medium and high-rent areas. Also, unemployment in the outer areas was about 3.5 times higher than in middle/higher rent areas.

The substantial differences in the circumstances of households in low rent areas as compared to households in medium and high rent areas, illustrated in Table 6.1, meant that households in the low rent areas had far greater levels of financial stress. In response to the question, "Over the past year, have any of the following happened to you/your household because of a shortage of money?", almost two thirds (63%) of tenants in low rent areas experienced at least one of the eight financial stress indicators listed in Fig. 6.1 below compared to 32% in the middle and inner areas.

One in seven renters in the low-rent outer areas said that they had had to forego meals and over a third had sought financial help from friends or family and had trouble paying utility bills on time; whereas only one in 25 renters in the medium and high rent areas said that they went without meals and one in ten had had trouble paying utility bills on time. Interestingly, one in six renters in medium/high rent areas had sought financial help from friends or family.

Figure 6.2 illustrates that a large proportion of tenants in low rent areas experienced multiple forms of financial stress, with 29% reporting more than three financial stress indicators and one in five reporting four or more. In contrast, in high and medium rent areas one in ten renters had three or more financial stress indicators and 6%

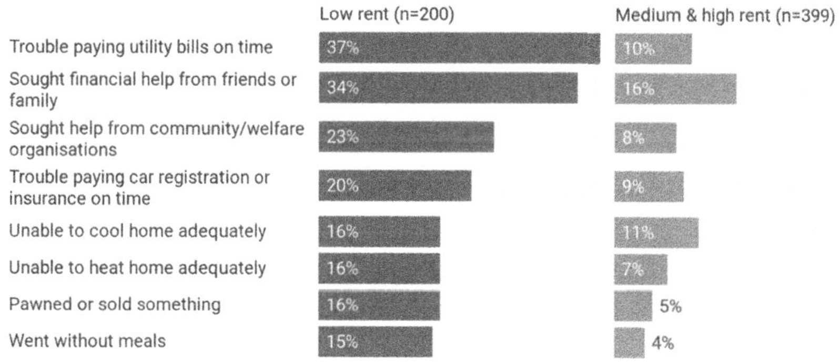

Fig. 6.1 Financial stress indicators by rent area (*Source* Authors' survey 2015)

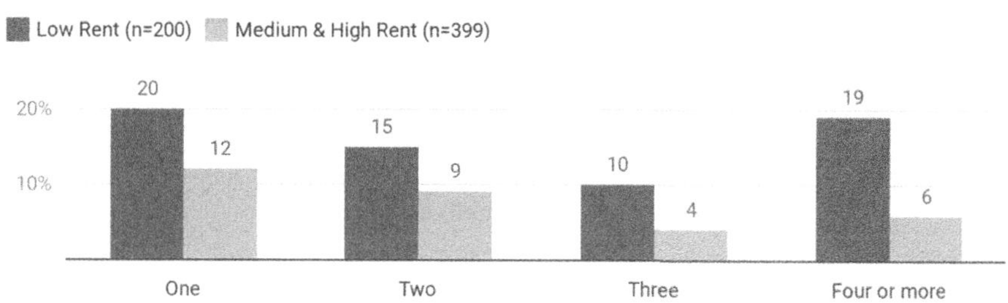

Fig. 6.2 Spread of financial stress indicators

had four or more. The experience of multiple and different forms of financial stress over time is likely to have major effects on the health and wellbeing of private renter household members.

Private Renters Dependent on Government Benefits

An important finding from our survey is that tenants reliant on government benefits irrespective of type of rental market area were likely to suffer from multiple indicators of financial stress. More than a third (37%) had recently experienced four or more of the financial stress indicators. Alarmingly, income poverty had resulted in 26% going without meals. Over a quarter (27%) of households where a household member was either looking for work, out of the work-force or retired, had experienced four or more forms of financial stress. Strikingly, this was true for only 5% of households where at least one person was in full-time employment.

The figures tell only a part of the story. The interviews we conducted with members of private renter households in receipt of government benefits gave us a much deeper and nuanced understanding of the effects of rental stress. Those interviewed were invariably having to use a considerable proportion of their income to pay for their accommodation. Sylvia, in Sydney's outer suburbs, was barely managing on her sole source of income—the government's parenting payment[6] and RA.

> I've got a water bill that's meant to be paid by today. It is only $75, but I paid the rest of the $180 off the electricity bill yesterday, so it has left me a little bit short. I've only got like $110 to get me though for the next week. Hopefully his dad will come through and give me some money next week … but yeah, so my water bills' going to be late …

Her fridge was not working, but she was unable to replace it; she had no savings and was unable to access credit:

> Yeah, I have to buy a new fridge … I tried to get one a couple of weeks ago, but my finances are shit cos I didn't pay an AGL [energy company] bill … so now I've got a bad credit rating cos I didn't finish paying the last $75 off. I can borrow through Cash Stop. I can get $5,000 through them, but the interest is so high, so I'm just going to, I'll save up some money somehow and I'll just go and get $600[7] from Cash Stop and I'll pay the rest in cash and get a new fridge.

Pam was also a single parent in Sydney's outer suburbs. Having received a notice to vacate, she was extremely anxious that she and her five children could find themselves homeless:

> Yeah, we got [90 days] notice, but still trying to you know find somewhere you can [afford] … For a while there I was thinking we'll be out on the street. It was so hard.

---

[6]In January 2020, the Parenting Payment was a maximum of $430 a week.

[7]In July 2020, Cash Stop's advertised that a loan of $600 over 4 months would cost $816 and over a year, $1008.

Historically in Australia the unemployment benefit has been far lower than all other government benefits.[8] Since the dissolution of her marriage, Michaela (57) had been reliant on private rental. When interviewed, she had been renting the same free-standing house in Sydney's outer suburbs for 16 years. She had lost her job two years prior to the interview due to poor health. Despite this, she had been denied the Disability Support pension (DSP) and was therefore forced to rely on Newstart and RA. Although her rent was very reasonable for Sydney, it was impossible for her to cover essential costs. Fortunately, she received some support from her daughter. When asked if it would be difficult to manage if not for her daughter, she responded,

> Very much so because my benefit is $650 a fortnight and the rent is $570 [a fortnight] which would leave like $80. I have electricity, I have gas, food you know … Right now, I'm with Job Centre Australia. They're trying to find me work that I will be able to do because I just can't manage on you know that money [Newstart]. It's terrible, but I mean that's what the payment is, so you have to deal with it, don't you?

As Michaela mentioned, her rent, $285 a week,[9] was very reasonable for the area, and she felt relatively fortunate despite her rent accounting for about 90% of her regular income:

> I thought I was being hard done by when they put my rent up, but when I look at what properties are going for around the area and I see their rents around $400, $500, I guess I'm lucky. It just seemed a lot to me because I'm you know on the Centrelink[10] benefit and it takes the majority of my money. My daughter gives me money to buy food and do all that, pay bills …

Recently her daughter had moved out and could no longer assist her. She was extremely worried about managing without her and the possibility of finding herself homeless:

> I want a job to get out of this rut with no money and you know [it's] hard to buy food and pay my bills. My electricity bill is $1800 at the moment. I can't pay it you know. I had a family living with me that have just recently moved on and got their own place and they can't afford to give me money for that now cos they've got to pay you know $400 and something a week rent. I'm stuck with the power bill. I don't have the money to pay that. I rang up Energy Australia [energy utility] and got a payment plan, staying connected plan. But the fact of the matter is the last three payments I couldn't make that because I didn't have the money to pay that either. So god only knows what's going to happen to me. I'm struggling right now financially and trying to get ahead … I'm thinking, I'm going to get in trouble here … I've got no money coming in and the power bill, the gas bill haven't been paid.

Sadly, Michaela's financial precarity meant that she was having to make decisions around what essentials to cut:

---

[8]In June 2019, the basic Newstart payment was $278 a week, whereas the basic Disability Support Pension (DSP) and the Age Pension rate was $422 a week. Michaela had been assessed as fit to work and deemed ineligible for the DSP. As mentioned, in March 2020, in response to the massive increase in unemployment due to the pandemic, the unemployment benefit was increased to $550 a week. At the end of March 2021, the unemployment supplement related to the Covid-19 pandemic was scrapped and the benefit, now called JobSeeeker, was increased by $25 a week to $310.40 for a single person.

[9]Note that the median rent for outer Sydney in June 2015 (all property sizes) was $430 per week (NSW Government Rent and Sales report database).

[10]Centrelink is the government agency that administers social security.

> So the other thing I have, I have a communication problem with my family because I don't have the money to buy credit for my phone because that's $30 for the phone. So the phone's $30, no food. So I buy my food instead of buying phone credit.

Like Michaela, Ingrid (low-rent, Melbourne) was worried about her energy bill. She was reliant on the DSP and severely restricted her use of heating:

> If I use that [big heater] my whole pension will go. You know, I usually don't use a heater at all. I have a small heater when I feel really cold I use it … But that big one, it's an old-fashioned one, so … my pension also won't remain if I've got to use that. So I dress up in a lot of clothes, two or three pairs of socks, and that's how I live.

Ill-health had forced Nigel (outer suburbs, Sydney) out of employment. He had been receiving workers' compensation for a work injury, but at the time of the interview was reliant on Newstart and CRA. The only way he was able to pay the rent and purchase necessities was with the help of friends:

> I've now gone from work to an insurance [workers compensation] that was covering me. Now the insurance stopped covering me. Now [that] I'm unemployed, I'm getting $661 a fortnight. My rent is $660.[11] So if it wasn't for friends you know …

Not surprisingly he was finding everyday life extremely difficult:

> Stress, yes, like stress is gone beyond a joke. It is not even the word for it. You don't know what's going to happen the next day … I'm just worried about where, how I'm going to survive. I've got the money every fortnight for rent, but that's all I've got.

He was desperately trying to access public housing.

When interviewed, Gail was on the Age Pension and living in social housing in Sydney. However, for several years in her fifties, she had been reliant on Newstart. She recounted how her lack of financial resources meant that for a period she was forced to reside in a boarding house and cut back on necessities. Her diet was a major concern:

> I'd buy frozen stuff because cooking was too expensive. I would buy frozen stuff and fruit and then I wouldn't be having any vegetables with it you know. I would have salad every now and again … Very rarely could you get into the kitchen to organise yourself to prepare something or it'd be taken out of the fridge before you got it. This was in the shared accommodation … The way I used to eat was horrendous, horrific.

The capacity of tenants on government benefits to cope with any rent increase is extremely limited. Raelene was living by herself in outer Melbourne and reliant on the DSP. She recounted how she was forced to move after the house she was living in was sold and the new owner increased her rent by $50 a week:

> They put it up about an extra $50 a week from what I was paying, and that's why I told the new owner, I said, "Look I'm sorry. I have to move because I can't afford to stay …"

[11] A relatively low rent for the area—see previous footnote.

Often households reliant on government benefits could only afford unsuitable accommodation and had to make sacrifices that affected their lives. Lenka (low rent, Melbourne) was a single parent and a full-time carer for her one daughter. She slept in the lounge, so that her three children could each have their own bedroom. She could not afford to move:

> I was here five years before we had our first rental increase. So comparatively, for what we've actually got, the cost is what keeps us here. Because if we were to go and have something of the same specifications … we'd be easily paying in excess of $300, and we can't afford that. So that's what keeps us here, because we're at least $40-odd under that per week, which makes a huge difference.

After her husband passed away, Amivi (low rent, Melbourne, reliant on DSP) decided she had to move. However, she was only able to afford a one-bedroom apartment which made it difficult for her to host visitors.

> If I rented two bedrooms, I don't have money enough probably. My aunt comes to stay with me … She often comes to me … when she's sick … So I would like to have two bedrooms. It's good [for] the old lady to have another one [bedroom] or my sisters or brothers come from Darwin. But, I think it's hard for me to pay [the rent for a two-bedroom apartment], especially in this area.

Patsy (low rent, Melbourne) was also reliant on the DSP and had been sharing with three people for seven years. She was in her mid-forties and her marriage had ended several years prior. Sharing not only lowered her rent considerably, but she also enjoyed the company of her house-mates.

> We share … It's four people who lives in the house … It's quite expensive if you sort of do it [rent] solo … With four people you share all the expenses. … It's cheaper and it's not only that, it's more. You've got someone to talk to … It's good because if something happens they know where you are and you know, they can help you.

While it worked for Patsy, sharing a house with others to lower the rent was not an option for others.

Renters Reliant on the Government Age Pension

Older renters reliant on the government Age Pension (see page 72 for a brief discussion of the government Age Pension) are particularly vulnerable (Morris, 2016). Health conditions may call for expenditure not necessarily covered by Medicare.[12] Also, their capacity to relocate in the event of a rent increase or end of tenancy notification, is often limited by a lack of internet access or a vehicle to look for alternative properties. Frailty may also hamper their capacity to relocate (see Bates et al., 2019). They are usually extremely resistant to sharing their accommodation to cut costs.

[12] Medicare is the federal government health system. A person on the Age Pension would be able to obtain most medical procedures without having to pay. However, there are some items that are not covered, for example physiotherapy.

Many of the older renters interviewed were battling to purchase basic necessities and their capacity to engage with the world was severely circumscribed. Colin (71) lived alone in the outer suburbs of Sydney. He was struggling with everyday living costs:

> It is pretty much living from I could say, fortnight to fortnight.[13] As you can see with this rent increase now, I think it's [the pension] is about almost say $800; … $520 a fortnight it goes to rent … Centrelink already takes $50 for my electricity so that's gone already. I had another son staying here and he left me with quite a big electricity bill … He left me with a bill of about $1,000. This is about more than a year ago … [Another] $50 has got to go off to the TV marketing which will pay for that pressure cooker … At the moment I owe the chemist about $76 and it has been going on for two months and I haven't had the money to pay it and she's patient. She just sent a letter, "This account is overdue" … I would like to pay my way and, you see, I feel guilty because sometimes I can let go on some extravagance and then find it's either feed myself or pay the chemist. I just run short.

He had a car which he viewed as essential. Public transport in his neighbourhood is poor and having a car greatly facilitated shopping. He also used it to go fishing. However, he was battling to keep the car on the road.

> And you were talking about what would I do if the rent went up any more? I'd have to consider getting rid of the car … You cannot go about with a car uninsured … I mean one's got to eat whatever so I would … I'd have to sell the car.

The precarious financial situation of older renters had an impact on their physical and mental health. After having to move from her daughter's home into the PRS, Carol's health deteriorated:

> My situation makes me feel lonely. My blood pressure is constantly up. Like it is all this worry … but I'm trying to not to give up, yeah.

Fran's (72) situation was desperate. A widower, she lived alone in a high-rent area in Sydney so as to be close to her family. Her rent accounted for almost all of her Age Pension and she was only able to get by because her daughter covered her essential costs. Her depression appeared to be linked to her dire financial situation:

> But I do think when it gets to the stage where they can't look after the elderly people you should be able to give them Nembutal [euthanasia drug] … I do think that when it gets to the stage where the Age Pension doesn't even cover your net, I do think you should be entitled to take something.

Although her situation was not as acute as Fran's, Glenda (70) was also battling. She lived by herself in Sydney's outer suburbs:

> See I do go out and I volunteer. I might go out four days, well that's $20 out of my pension every fortnight. So I've had to really watch [my money]. Do you need to go out today? Do you need to go on the train? … It colours every aspect of your life. Your entertainment, your physical [health] … And as you get older you do; I want to look after myself. I don't want to be a burden. So I do try and, a friend gave me a juicer so I have a carrot juice every day and carrots are quite cheap - 99 cents for a couple of kilos … But yes, I have had days where if I had a light bill or a phone bill … I'll eat baked beans. Baked beans are really good. They're nutritious and I shop at Aldi now … They have tins of baked beans for 19 cents, so I stock up with those …

[13]The Age Pension is paid every two weeks.

She was unable to save:

> And I always try to keep at least $20. If I've got $20 by the next Monday I'm doing it good and I try to keep that because it's not so depressing. It is depressing, it is. We shouldn't live for money, but that's what people want from us … What I do at Christmas, I go and get the $500 that Centrelink [the government agency responsible for organising pension payments] allows you to have, and you pay it off. And that's how I buy Christmas presents.

Any major expense is a major setback for private renters surviving on very low incomes. Charles (82) was having to pay the bank almost half his pension after borrowing money for his wife's funeral:

> I had to borrow money because I was just living on the pension and I had to borrow money off the bank for the funeral and everything like that. So I'm still paying that off which hurts a lot cos it takes half of me pension … I paid them last week … I've got nothing this week. So you just got to watch what you do. But I got good mates, they help me out.

Even couples were struggling. Cherie (77) and her husband (80) who had been home owners (see Chapter 4, page 78) lived from pension payment to pension payment. There was no possibility of saving:

> Everything seems to be covered with our pensions going in and the rent is being paid, that comes out of our bank, but there's not much left … We don't have a computer or anything like that. We couldn't afford it. Thinking about the electricity running things, I don't even have a mobile phone and we don't have a lot of household utilities … I [used to have] my hair cut once a month and I had it done today and that's the first time in four months that my hair has been cut and I cut my husband's myself.

Despite having around $250,000 in savings, Tony (66) and his wife (65) were highly stressed about their situation. They were renting a house on the Central Coast and constantly weighing up whether to buy a home or continue renting. They were concerned that by continuously having to dip into their savings to cover living costs, any hope of home ownership would eventually disappear:

> The only problem is like we've got a bit of cash, but we will eventually go through that. The pension we're finding, we can't quite live on. Yeah, so I guess we don't know what the answer is … Well, it's [the stress] huge, yeah. And we talk about it [purchasing a home or renting], my wife and I, talk about it almost daily. She looks at houses in some pretty ordinary areas … on the Central Coast[14] and some of them are quite rough areas. Something that we can afford. Yeah, so it's not an option we are comfortable with, but while that would tie up our money at least we'd have the asset. So it is a quandary … So if you owned your own home, I mean you're not spending money on rent. You haven't got that big payment every week. … It's not a lot of money that we're short, but we are short.

If a person on the Age Pension is a smoker their private rental options are severely reduced. Their expenditure on cigarettes means they do not have the finances to afford conventional rental accommodation. Steve, reliant on the Age Pension, was a heavy smoker. He had no furniture and was forced to rent in boarding houses or pubs. He could not afford to recharge his mobile phone:

---

[14]The Central Coast is about 80 kilometres from Sydney. Its house prices are substantially lower than Sydney house prices.

> I haven't recharged it for 18 months. I give people the phone number and they can ring me, but I can't ring them. I've got to go with the local phone box. Either that or borrow one ... And one thing with mobiles, I mean the minimum recharge you can get is $30. That's a whack out of somebody's pension.

Some older renters had been fortunate. They had found adequate accommodation for a reasonable rent and were coping. This was more likely in regional areas. Lorraine (68) lived alone in regional New South Wales and was paying $150 a week. She also earned a small amount cleaning a neighbour's apartment. She was frugal, but was able to engage in a range of activities. When asked if "she had to be very careful in terms of expenditure", she responded,

> Not really. If I want something, ... if I think well, I really want that, I'll go without something else ... Yes, I go out on Friday night. It is only to the local club, but it is very handy. There's a community you know, community of people that I've managed to meet [that] I'm friends with. I have always got wine and beer in the fridge ... I mean I can't go drinking French champagne, but if I want a bottle of wine I can go and buy it, ... You know if I want a prime cut of meat I can go and get it. I can't do it every night of the week.

When interviewed Natalie (72) had recently accessed social housing. When asked how the move from the PRS into social housing had changed her life, she eloquently reflected on how the stress she constantly experienced ended once she secured affordable, secure housing:

> Well it has changed because the stress has simply fallen off my shoulders ... It has been wonderful. ... I probably wasn't fully aware of how stressed I really was and just how every day was [about] how much cash have I still got in my wallet? What do I need to get with that cash, and every day was a little list on my desk with everything I needed, not what I wanted. ... And it just kind of like, just got to the stage where I got so stressed over it, I was wondering [whether] the next rent rise that's me out on the street ... And I even thought, I'm doing the right thing getting out there, putting all my stuff in the middle of the road and getting the television stations there and making an issue of it seriously. ... It reduces your capacity for even the simplest of things which we all, when we are working with good money coming in, just simply take for granted I think the fact that I can now, if I want to, I can go into a shop like the reject shop which I love because it has got all those good things that I like and can enjoy and if I want stationary I can go in there ... I never bought envelopes because I couldn't afford them ... So now I can go and buy envelopes if I want ... I can talk to you for half-an-hour on that phone without me worrying about it. That's another thing is that I can phone you up and I don't have to say, "I'm sorry, the credit's going to run out in a minute". It isn't [any longer] cos I've got all that money there [so] if I want to talk for half-an-hour, I can.

Employed Renters

Our survey of renters in Sydney and Melbourne indicated that renters in employment were significantly more likely to find paying the rent "very easy" or "quite easy" compared to renters reliant on a government benefits, as shown in Table 6.2. One in five wage or salary earners said that they found it not easy or not at all easy to pay the rent, compared to half of private renters reliant on government benefits.

Table 6.2 How easy does your household find it to afford the rent payments? (%)

	Very easy (n = 125) %	Quite easy (n = 324) %	Not easy (n = 126) %	Not at all easy (n = 25) %
Wages or salaries	22	57	18	3
Self-funded retiree	20	80	0	0
State pensions or benefits (excluding age pension)	7	43	40	10
Age Pension	13	46	38	4
Other	31	45	16	9
Total	21	54	21	4

Source Authors' survey 2015

Households with Employed Members and Still Struggling

Although having employed household members certainly lessens the possibility of a household being in rental stress, it is no guarantee that paying the rent is stress-free. Among our interviewees, some households where one member was employed full-time were struggling financially—the rent was a major burden. Gina (low-rent, Sydney) was not working, however her husband was working full-time. They had two teenage daughters:

> And like we don't have credit cards or anything. Like everything we've got, we own. Like we don't have anything unnecessary. We try to avoid that, but you still find yourself, not scraping, but you know you've just got to watch what you do with your money ... Like it's hard and even when I do start working I can't see that we are going to be able to save a lot of money to still put money away. Like we'll try, but how many years is it going to take? You know what I mean. It is going to take a long time.

Winnie (low-rent, Sydney) stopped working after the birth of her daughter, leaving her partner as the household's sole breadwinner. She recounted how hard it was being dependent on one salary:

> I remember earlier in our marriage ... the rent would get paid, but we wouldn't eat. It used to be really bad back then ... I'd make sure Fred [her husband] would have something because he had to work, but myself and the little girl we sort of skimped you know.

Although their situation had improved over the years, she still felt vulnerable.

> [It's] a lot easier now. I mean, if we want to go to a concert or something like that we don't have to think we'll have to save for weeks to do it ... We can go and do it if we want to, but if we move and the rent goes up that might curtail that a bit. And you're supposed to get more comfortable as you get older, but in a lot of cases it doesn't [happen].

Some households with employed members endured over-crowded conditions to mitigate rental stress. Annchi lived with her husband, 21 year-old daughter and her mother in a two-bedroom apartment in a medium-rent area in Melbourne. She was working part-time and her husband full-time. When asked if she felt comfortable inviting friends over, she responded,

> Not any more … It's more because my daughter is getting, is growing, so we now change the lounge-room to be her bedroom, so that's why … we don't feel comfortable inviting [friends over].

She was concerned about the lack of space and resented the last rent increase, but felt that they could not afford to move to more spacious accommodation:

> Yeah, yeah, because that's also actually one [affordability] of the reasons why we couldn't move out. So like … when they increase it so much, we wanted to move out. We can't get a bigger place with a bit less rental price … I want more rooms for my family, especially because my daughter needs her own room, and I would love to also have a spare room so we can use it for a working office, or maybe when somebody comes over they can stay with us.

A single parent in a high paying public service job, Louise was renting in a high-rent area in Sydney. She had found an old semi to rent and had spent a fair amount of time and money making it pristine. Although she was coping with the "expensive rent", she was concerned about the future:

> It is a bit grim to be honest you know, so I've just thought … I'm going to have to you know put some money away and hopefully find some little hovel in the countryside you know to buy or rent when I'm living on my superannuation or whatever. Or maybe I'll have to use my superannuation for that, who knows.

Share Houses

Our survey found that one in five renter households in the selected areas of Sydney and Melbourne were share houses (group households where the adults were not related). The proportion was especially high in medium and high-rent areas where close to one in three rental households were share houses, whereas in low-rent areas only one in 25 was (Table 6.3).

Most tenants in share houses (85%) were under 35; 39% were under 25. It is likely that almost all of the under 25 group were students as were many of the 25–34 year-old grouping and were sharing to cut costs. A proportion of sharers were employed and not students and were likely sharing in order to afford the rent in more convenient and expensive locations. Andrew was single, employed full-time and sharing a house in a medium-rent area in Sydney. Sharing allowed him to rent a larger property in a convenient location. Despite sharing he was battling and contemplating looking for cheaper accommodation. His rent in 2015 was $380 a week:

> I think yeah, sort of between me, you and the wall behind you it's a bit of a struggle So from my perspective now I'm sort of thinking you know how much longer can I stay here for. Maybe I should go and look for something you know around the $200 mark a week … You just can't do the things that you want to do … Yeah, just sort of makes life a little bit difficult I suppose when you haven't got the money. You seem to just have enough money to cover all the essentials and hang on, I haven't got a life, I can't live. I can't afford the you know, can't afford to do this or that, so you've got to look for cheap forms of entertaining yourself and having a life.

Table 6.3 Which of the following best describes this household?

	Sole person ($n =$ 108) %	Couple ($n =$ 119) %	Couple with at least one dependent child ($n =$ 155) %	One parent with at least one dependent child ($n =$ 50) %	Single or couple with independent child(ren) (i.e. not living with parents) (n = 15) %	Group house (unrelated adult sharers) (n = 122) %	Other ($n =$ 30) %	Total %
High and medium rent areas	16	21	22	6	2	29	5	100
Low rent areas	23	17	33	14	5	4	6	100
Total	18	20	26	8	3	20	5	100

Source Authors' survey 2015

Rick was sharing in a medium-rent area in Melbourne. He appeared to be coping adequately:

> You earn your wages, live within your means. I don't live on credit, never have done. So it [renting] doesn't prevent me from doing anything really, no. Rent's number one. Do rent, one, and you've got a roof over your head. Pay your bills, you get electricity, you get water. Go shopping, you've got food … So if you've got all that then everything else just falls into place … I earn enough to pay my bills and pay for my rent. So yeah, it doesn't stop me doing anything. Oh, we'd all like to be rich wouldn't we?

Dual Income Households

For couples with both partners working full-time, rental stress is much less likely. Of the 129 households in our survey where there were two members working full-time, only 12% said it was not easy or not at all easy to pay the rent, whereas for the 233 households with only one person working full-time, 24% said it was not easy or not at all easy to pay the rent.

Nirmal (low-rent, Melbourne) and his wife were both in full-time work. They were having absolutely no problem paying the rent:

> At this point of time we don't have to compromise with living standards. We can eat whatever we want, and we can save as well. We've been able to save a fair bit of money staying in this house.

In a medium-rent area in Melbourne, Shirley and her sister were paying $1875 a month for a three-bedroom apartment. They had little problem affording the rent: "Yeah, but there's two people that are working [full-time], so it's not that bad".

A less common case was that of Amber and her husband who were living in a stunning five-bedroom home in a high-rent area in Sydney. They had left their high-flying jobs in the financial sector and put all their capital into their business. Their capacity to afford the rent, just over $2000 a week, was dependent on how well their business was doing:

> When we moved into this place our business was going a bit crazy and we sort of got all excited, but you know we're in a bigger place and then we had a bit of a bad run. A few things happened and so our business sort of had a bit of a bad patch. And it has taken us a while to recover from that. So initially this place was affordable and then it became a little bit of a stretch, but to a point our landlord has been very understanding. I think in this market, this sort of price range you get a few expats but not a lot of private Australians in that range because what we spend on rent would probably go to a mortgage. Our problem is that we don't have a deposit, so you know we realise we pay a lot in rent.

Can Comfortably Rent, but Cannot Buy

Although employed renters in medium and high-rent areas usually found their rent affordable most doubted that they would ever have the means to purchase a property—at least in that area. Ben was renting in a medium-rent area in Melbourne:

> Houses here are like $1.5 million now, so I couldn't buy here in my wildest dreams, but I can live here, so that's the advantage [of remaining as a tenant]. I can rent here and that's a big advantage ...

Hazel, her husband and two children lived in a free-standing four-bedroom house in Sydney. Her husband had a "good job" and they could afford the rent ($750 a week in December 2015), but could not contemplate purchasing a home in Sydney.

> Although we would really like to get something stable [and] we'd like to buy at some point, but there's no way we could afford to live in Sydney. There's no way we can get a deposit to buy a place because it's all so expensive. Yeah, and we've got part of a deposit but if we have to get 10 or 20% of $1.5 million you know, it's just unattainable.

Tomas was living with his partner, a dog and three cats (needed a backyard) in a medium-rent area in Sydney. He had also given up any notion of purchasing in Sydney:

> We have been priced out of the market for wanting a house with a backyard. Every little rundown shit-box has been renovated you know. Everybody is watching the DIY (do it yourself) shows and ...... so for us it's the Central Coast or southern highlands[15] you know and we're then adding an extra hour to our commute before we get started ... The old days where it's [renting] been a stop gap between your study, you might live in the city for a few years and then you save up and buy a place, they're gone. With the price that it is at the moment, once you're stuck in that [rental] trap it is a cycle that you can't get out of.

---

[15] The Central Coast is approximately 80 kilometres from Sydney and the Southern Highlands is 130 kilometres—a two-hour drive.

Conclusions

The PRS is certainly diverse in terms of tenants' household incomes and rent levels. Not surprisingly, private renters who are reliant on the Age Pension or other government benefits invariably experience rental stress with far-reaching implications. It meant that they were unable to lead a decent life. Amartya Sen defines a decent life in terms of people's capabilities—a person's capacity "to lead the kind of lives they value and have reason to value" (Sen, 1999, p. 18). When a person is having to use a considerable proportion of their income for rent, their capabilities are necessarily severely constrained. They simply do not have the opportunities to pursue what they value and their agency and choices are severely circumscribed. This lack of capability or what Sen calls "capability deprivation" has a major impact on wellbeing. Not only do they lack the necessary income to buy essentials, but, as we shall see in the next chapter (Chapter 7), they also had to contend with high levels of insecurity. For many of the renters reliant on government benefits the high levels of rental stress they experienced resulted not only in financial difficulties but also affected their health and wellbeing. They reported that they experienced severe psychological stress and, in some instances, appeared to be seriously depressed counting every cent and often running short of money prior to the next pension/benefit day.

In contrast, households where at least one member was employed full-time were usually able to cope with the rent. However, even some of these households were struggling especially in middle and higher rent areas. A large proportion of renters, especially in the younger age groups in middle and high rent areas, lessened the possibility of rental stress by choosing to share.

Households where both members were employed full-time rarely had difficulty paying for their accommodation. However, within these households there was much pessimism about the possibility of transitioning to home ownership in the future in the areas they were currently renting in. There was consensus that "graduation to home ownership" would be achievable only at the cost of leaving their suburb for a relatively remote location, if at all.

References

ABS (Australian Bureau of Statistics). (2019). *3236.0—Household and family projections, Australia, 2016 to 2041*. Canberra: ABS. https://www.abs.gov.au/ausstats/abs@.nsf/Latestproducts/3236.0Main%20Features42016%20to%202041?opendocument&tabname=Summary&prodno=3236.0&issue=2016%20to%202041&num=&view=.

ABS (Australian Bureau of Statistics). (2020). *62020.0 labour force, Australia, April 2020*. Canberra: ABS. https://www.abs.gov.au/AUSSTATS/abs@.nsf/Lookup/6202.0Main%20Features1Apr%202020.

AHURI Brief. (2019). *Understanding the 30:40 indicator of housing affordability stress*. Melbourne: AHURI (Australian Housing and Urban Research Institute Limited).

Anglicare Australia. (2020). *Rental affordability snapshot: National report 2020*. Sydney: Anglicare.

Baker, E., Mason, K., & Bentley, R. (2015). Measuring housing affordability: A longitudinal approach. *Urban Policy and Research, 33*(3), 275–290. https://doi.org/10.1080/08111146.2015.1034853.

Baker, E., Pham, N. T. A., Daniel, L., & Bentley, R. (2020). New evidence on mental health and housing affordability in cities: A quantile regression approach. *Cities, 96,* 1–7. https://doi.org/10.1016/j.cities.2019.102455.

Bates, L., Wiles, J., & Kearns, R. (2019). Precariously placed: Home, housing and wellbeing for older renters. *Health & Place, 58*(July), 1.9. https://doi.org/10.1016/j.healthplace.2019.102152.

Bentley, R. J., Pevalin, D., Bake, E., Mason, K., Reeves, A., & Beer, A. (2016). Housing affordability, tenure and mental health in Australia and the United Kingdom: A comparative panel analysis. *Housing Studies, 31*(2), 208–222.

Burke, T., Stone, M., & Ralston, L. (2011). *The residual income method: A new lens on housing affordability and market behaviour, No. 176.* Melbourne: AHURI.

Campbell, I., Parkinson, S., & Wood, G. (2014). *Underemployment and housing insecurity: An empirical analysis of HILDA data, No. 230.* Melbourne: AHURI (Australian Housing and Urban Research Limited). https://www.ahuri.edu.au/research/final-reports/230.

Herrick, H., & Di Bona, V. (2013). *The association of housing stress, health, chronic disease and health care resources: Results from the 2011 North Carolina BRFSS Survey.* Raleigh, NC: State Centre for Health Statistics.

Hulse, K., Reynolds, M., Nygaard, C., & Yates, J. (2019). *The supply of affordable private rental housing in Australian cities: Short-term and longer-term changes.* Melbourne: AHURI (Australian Housing and Urban Research Limited).

Mallett, S., Bentley, R., Baker, E., Mason, K., Key, D., Kolar, V., & Krnjacki, L. (2011). *Precarious housing and health inequalities: What are the links?* Melbourne: University of Melbourne, Hanover Welfare Services, University of Adelaide & Melbourne City Mission.

Melbourne Institute. (2018). *Poverty lines: Australia, March quarter.* Melbourne: Applied Economic & Social Research, Melbourne Institute.

Metzler, R., & Schwartz, A. (2016). Housing affordability and health: Evidence from New York City. *Housing Policy Debate, 26*(1), 80–104.

Morris, A. (2016). *The Australian dream: Housing experiences of older Australians.* Melbourne: CSIRO Publishing.

Morris, A. (2018). Housing tenure and the health of older Australians dependant on the age pension for their income. *Housing Studies, 18*(1), 77–95.

Nepal, D., Tanton, R., & Harding, A. (2010). Measuring housing stress: How much do definitions matter? *Urban Policy and Research, 28*(2), 211–224. https://doi.org/10.1080/08111141003797454.

Padley, M., & Marshall, L. (2019). Defining and measuring housing affordability using the Minimum Income Standard. *Housing Studies, 34*(8), 1307–1329. https://doi.org/10.1080/02673037.2018.1538447.

Pawson, H., Milligan, V., & Yates, J. (2020). *Housing policy in Australia: A case for system reform.* Singapore: Palgrave.

Productivity Commission. (2019). *Vulnerable private renters: Evidence and options.* Canberra: Australian Government.

Robinson, E., & Adams, R. (2008). *Housing stress and the mental health and wellbeing of families.* Canberra: Australian Government.

Rosier, K., & McDonald, M. (2011). *The relationship between transport and disadvantage in Australia.* Canberra: Australian Institute of Family Studies, Australian Government.

Rowley, S., & Ong, R. (2012). *Housing affordability, housing stress and household wellbeing in Australia, No. 192.* Melbourne: AHURI (Australian Housing and Urban Research Institute Limited).

Rowley, S., Ong, R., & Haffner, M. (2015). Bridging the gap between housing stress and financial stress: The case of Australia. *Housing Studies, 30*(3), 473–490.

Saunders, P., & Bedford, M. (2018). New minimum health living budget standards for low paid and unemployed Australians. *The Economic and Labour Relations Review, 29*(3), 273–288.
Sen, A. (1999). *Development as freedom*. Oxford: Oxford University Press.
SGS Economics & Planning. (2019). *Rental Affordability Index*. Canberra: National Shelter, Community Sector Banking, Independent Insight & Brotherhood St Laurence.
Stone, M. E. (2006). What is housing affordability? The case for the residualism approach. *Housing Policy Debate, 17*(1), 151–184.
Sweet, E., Nandi, A., Adam, E. K., & McDade, T. W. (2013). The high price of debt: Household financial debt and its impact on mental and physical health. *Social Science and Medicine, 91*, 94–100.
Taylor, M. P., Pevalin, D. J., & Todd, J. (2007). The psychological costs of unsustainable housing commitments. *Psychological Medicine, 37*, 1027–1036.
Whelan, S., & Parkinson, S. (2017). *Housing tenure, mobility and labour market behaviour, No. 280*. Melbourne: AHURI (Australian Housing and Urban Research Institute Limited).
Yates, J., & Gabriel, M. (2006). *Housing affordability in Australia: Housing affordability for low income Australians, Research Paper No. 3*. Melbourne: AHURI (Australian Housing and Urban Research Institute Limited).
Yates, J., & Milligan, V. (2007). *Housing affordability: A 21st century problem, No. 105*. Melbourne: AHURI (Australian Housing and Urban Research Institute Limited).

Chapter 7
Renting and Insecurity

Abstract Light regulation of the PRS means that private renters on short fixed term leases or periodic tenancies can be required to leave their home at short notice, typically when the property is being sold or if the landlord or their family wants to live in the property. In most Australian states they can also be given notice to leave without any stated grounds. The law also allows for regular increases in rents to "market levels" without any cap on the increase. Landlord freedoms to end tenancies and/or raise rent can make continued tenancy difficult or impossible. The chapter investigates tenants' experiences of insecurity in their housing situation as legal insecurity does not necessarily translate into *de facto* insecurity. It also examines perceptions of insecurity which can differ markedly. The chapter finds that while private renters develop some strategies to adapt to their situation on a daily basis such that insecurity is often only "at the back of the mind", all perceive lack of control over their housing futures. The capacity of low-income tenants to deal with a rent increase or notice to vacate is often very different to the capacity of medium and higher income tenants.

Introduction

We saw in Chapter 1 that Australia began to adopt regulation of landlord-tenant relations for its highly urbanised society in the late 1970s. Despite successive state government changes to details of residential tenancies legislation since then, Chapter 2 outlined how this legislation remains relatively weak in terms of consumer rights and protections compared to countries in Europe and elsewhere (Hulse et al., 2011; Martin et al., 2018). Regulation of tenancies provides the institutional framework for private renting along with the housing and other public policies considered in Chapter 3.

Previous chapters have suggested, however, that tenants' experiences of insecurity in the PRS is also shaped by a variety of other factors which, in combination, affect their housing pathways (Chapter 4), the extent to which they are able to make a home in their rented property (Chapter 5); and the sometimes pernicious effects of financial stress in paying rent from low incomes (Chapter 6). These contribute

A. Morris et al., *The Private Rental Sector in Australia*,
https://doi.org/10.1007/978-981-33-6672-5_7

to what has been called de facto housing insecurity—experiences of insecurity in everyday life (Fitzpatrick & Pawson, 2014). In addition, how PRS tenants perceive insecurity (*perceptual* insecurity) (Hulse & Milligan, 2014) may vary across groups as well as for different individuals. This chapter seeks to understand private renters' experiences and perceptions, taking this broader view of insecurity.

The chapter proceeds as follows. Firstly, it unpacks some of the interrelated dimensions which contribute to housing insecurity. Secondly, we consider private tenants' experiences of housing insecurity before, thirdly, examining tenants' perceptions of insecurity. In so doing, we draw primarily on in-depth interviews with long-term tenants (10 plus years) and older tenants reliant on the government Age Pension, for whom the cumulative effects of the dimensions of housing insecurity could be expected to be most apparent.

The Dimensions of Housing Insecurity

Housing insecurity is a complex concept because it is multi-dimensional. Australian research on the topic has identified some of these dimensions: unchosen housing moves; housing instability (not knowing whether and when one has to move); lack of privacy, feeling unsafe, lack of belonging and lack of physical comfort (Hulse & Saugeres, 2008; Morris et al., 2017). A recent review of US research on housing insecurity confirms many of these albeit using different terminology, but adds, inadequate housing quality, homelessness, neighbourhood quality and overcrowding (Leopold et al., 2016, pp. 3–4). The key point from these studies is that each of these dimensions is often identified and measured separately but it is the interrelation between them that comprises housing insecurity. Thus, for example, housing instability may be associated with a lack of belonging as private renters may feel excluded from a community that they may have to exit at short notice. In another example, lack of physical comfort in rental accommodation with a low level of amenity or in poor condition may be associated with feeling unsafe.

Housing insecurity is experienced differently by different groups of people since tenant perceptions will be affected by varying expectations and tolerance levels. For example, older people and people with disabilities may perceive it differently to younger working people due to the additional difficulties the former may face in seeking alternative rental accommodation at short notice (see Morris, 2016). There are also individual differences in the perception of housing insecurity—feeling insecure—based on past experiences and future expectations. In this context, an under-researched area is how private renters use their agency to deal with what appears to be a high level of legal insecurity. We might also expect that experience of insecurity would have cumulative effects on perceptions over the longer term. To investigate these issues in detail, we focus on LTRs and older tenants' experiences and perceptions in this chapter.

Legal Security—Negotiated Through Everyday Practices

Especially as framed within the Anglophone country context, private renting is conventionally seen as providing weak "security of tenure" (Hulse et al. 2011; Martin et al. 2018) usually in comparison with home ownership. Important regulatory weakness highlighted by reviews of Australian legislation (Blunden & Martin, 2004; NATO et al., 2010) and that likely contribute to PRS insecurity, have been outlined in Chapter 2. However, although widely used, security of tenure is actually rather a vague concept beyond the legal terms and conditions of tenancy (Hulse & Milligan, 2014).

Legal provisions specify the rights and responsibilities of landlords and tenants, but these do not exist in a vacuum. Landlord-tenant relations depend on the understanding and practices of many small-scale landlords, the real estate agents they employ, and tenants themselves. They are forged through a myriad of transactions by 2.1 million people who own or part-own a rental property (ATO, 2018); 2.3 m private renter households (ABS, 2019) and about 35,000 real estate service businesses (ABS 2013).

Landlords who manage rental housing directly are often amateur property managers who may be unfamiliar with legal provisions and as a result their management practices may not always be compliant with legislative requirements (Hulse et al., 2018a). Managing agents represent landlords but they are also increasingly reliant on income from managing rental properties to generate income to support their businesses with such income generally related to rents charged and tenancy turnover (Hulse et al., 2018b). Tenants, on the other hand, will develop their own coping practices in the context of legal insecurity. For example, they may avoid requesting repairs because of fear that this will trigger a rent increase. In another example, in a regulatory context where pet ownership is allowed only at a landlord's discretion, renters with companion animals experience insecurity in knowing that they will find it more difficulty to find a new home if their current tenancy (Power 2017).

Landlord-tenant relations are also shaped by cultural norms around renting. For example, in the State of Victoria residential tenancies legislation enables fixed term leases of up to five years duration; however, landlords/agents routinely offer 12-month leases as standard and prospective tenants do not ask for longer leases. This appears to be a matter of cultural practice not regulation with neither landlords nor tenants keen to commit to longer term binding contracts. Landlords may see their property primarily as a capital asset, ideally capable of liquidation at short notice. Tenants, on the other hand may prioritise their ability to move for personal or employment reasons.

De facto Security

Housing insecurity has other dimensions beyond the legal relationship between landlords and tenants. Perhaps the best recognized and most widely researched of these is 'affordability' which depends on two factors - rents relative to household incomes.

Unaffordable rents, or rents which become unaffordable relative to incomes, will affect security for renters as discussed in Chapter 6. These experiences should be seen in the context of longer-term changes in supply, such as the increasing shortage of PRS housing affordable to very low-income households since 1996 (Hulse et al., 2019) and the effects of competition from an increasing number of middle and higher income tenants, which affects the availability of affordable rentals for low-income populations (Hulse et al., 2019). The other side of the affordability problem is income uncertainty. Labour market changes such as an increase in casual and contract work, unemployment, underemployment and zero hours contracts have made household income increasingly volatile and difficult to predict (Campbell & Burgess, 2018). Changes in income can also be precipitated by other types of disruptive life events such as family or relationship breakdown, domestic and family violence, or the onset of mental or physical ill-health.

Research has also highlighted the importance of non-financial factors, the so-called 'psycho-social' dimensions of housing insecurity. Interestingly, most of the research on this topic focuses on home ownership rather than renting and associates home ownership with a long list of psycho-social factors that contribute to high levels of housing security including: autonomy, privacy, control over one's own circumstances, "ontological security" and life satisfaction (Dupuis & Thorns, 1998; Kearns et al., 2000; Hiscock et al., 2001; Morris, 2016, 2018).

In contrast, specific research into private renting and the psycho-social dimensions of housing insecurity is limited and patchy (Hulse & Milligan, 2014, p. 18) although there is starting to be some research into this area internationally (e.g. Soatia et al., 2020) and it is an area that will undoubtedly receive more attention in the future due to the effects of the COVID-19 pandemic of 2020–2021. Some research posits links between insecurity and physical and mental health, social connectedness and well-being. For example, recent research (Morris, 2018) highlights the constant anxiety experienced by some older tenants about the possibility of an untenable rent increase or a forced move. Stress, poor self-identity, loneliness and depression may result (Morris, 2018). In their work with female private tenants, many with children, Hulse and Saugeres (2008) reported similar security worries, in some cases affecting health and wellbeing. A key theme in these accounts is lack of or loss of control over current and future housing circumstances. Feelings of safety and control over one's life in a context of reliability and constancy of life's daily routines provides a high degree of ontological security (Webb, 2018). This refers to a person's confidence in their self-identity and the constancy of their social and material environment. As such it is profoundly important to health and wellbeing.

Perceptual Insecurity

Perceptions are critical to an understanding of housing insecurity. *Perceptual* insecurity refers to a lack of a sense of security that a private tenant (in this case) may have about their housing situation. People may be anxious about the possibility of losing their tenancy whether the risk of a forced move is objectively high or not. Alternatively, they may feel secure in their housing even if the legal basis of their occupancy is limited (Hulse & Milligan, 2014). This is perhaps why research on tenants enjoying limited *de jure* security of tenure found that this did not necessarily translate into high levels of perceptual insecurity. Rather, many said that they had choice over how long they could stay in the dwelling; expressed a feeling of control over their tenancy arrangements and considered that the dwelling and location was appropriate to them (Minnery et al., 2003). This work suggests diverse perceptions of insecurity between groups of people and between individuals.

Apart from Minnery's work in Queensland Australia, differences in perceptual insecurity among private renters has been little studied although there are some signs that this is changing (e.g. Soatia et al., 2020). Some relevant insights are provided in a recent study of social housing tenant perceptions of the replacement of lifelong tenancies by fixed term tenancy contracts. According to their perceptions of this change, respondents were classed as the unaware, the unconcerned, or the anxious (Fitzpatrick & Watts, 2017, pp. 10–12), indicating that how people in similar circumstances perceive their [in]security is not predictable and can vary substantially.

To sum up this section on the dimensions of housing insecurity, the landlord-tenant relationship at the heart of private rental experience is a legal one, but it is more complex than this. It is also a power relationship which occurs in the context of different rental market contexts, develops through day to day practices, and is suffused with cultural norms about renting, being a tenant and being a landlord. Cultural norms are embedded in and transferred through the language that we use: we own a home but rent a house. In the next section, we examine how these factors interact to provide PRS tenants' experiences of housing insecurity.

Legal Security: Fixed Term Leases and Periodic Tenancies

Our survey of 600 private renters in Sydney and Melbourne indicated a clear difference between longer term and other renters in terms of their current lease arrangements (Pawson et al., 2017). Long term renters (10 plus years renting) were almost equally split between those who had a current fixed term lease (usually 6 or 12 months) and those who were on a periodic tenancy. This latter arrangement comes into play once a fixed term lease ends and is a rolling weekly or, more usually, monthly arrangement without a specified end date. In contrast almost two thirds of those renting for less 10 years had a current fixed term lease with a specified end date. Only a small number of respondents were uncertain about their current lease arrangement.

Longer-term tenants on fixed term leases saw advantages in terms of knowing where they would be living for the next 6 or 12 months. For example, Sophie was in her mid-30s living with partner and infant child in an inner Sydney suburb. She had wanted a wanted a fixed-term lease for greater security:

> When we moved in here I took a 12-month lease rather than a six month for the security for him [the baby]. I didn't want to have to move again in six months with a small baby and probably that would prompt me to sign another lease this time just … week to week so that cos having to move is like it was hard enough when he was four months old. I can't imagine doing it now that he's nearly 15 months old. It would be harder because he knows this place and space and he's really settled here.

Other tenants preferred shorter leases after the initial lease period has ended to give them greater flexibility. Rob, an older tenant who lived in Sydney, was one of these. He preferred a shorter lease to give him more options if his circumstances improved.

> I've got a 12-month lease and its variable you know. I can extend it if I want to for another 12 months, but what I normally do is take it on six months extension so if I do win $20 million lottery next week I haven't got so much money to pay to break the lease.

Some of the long-term renters had worked out, however, that renewing a fixed-term lease typically generated a rent increase unlike a periodic tenancy which went 'under the radar' without clear review points for resetting the rent. Paul was aged about 50 and had undergone a relationship break up. He lived with another adult in a middle-rent suburb of Melbourne and understood the thinking behind this practice.

> I have a year by year lease. Because I've been here for a while, sometimes they don't bother to renew it. It just keeps going on and then we'll sign another one when they want to put up the rent, if they want to put up the rent of something, so it tends to be a year lease.

Many long-term renters, however, appeared to be on a periodic tenancy entirely by default. Faith who lived by herself in a middle Melbourne suburb, argued that there were both advantages and disadvantages of a fixed-term lease. She had been living in the same place for 13 years:

> Well, I haven't actually signed a lease since the first year or two, and so it's just a rolling month-by-month thing. So in some ways, yeah, if I signed a lease, well, they couldn't kick me out until the end of that lease but, by the same token, if I wanted to leave I could leave but I would have to pay to the end of the lease. So it goes both ways.

Gina and family in an outer Sydney suburb were on a weekly periodic tenancy. She had worked out that this provided greater flexibility through the relevant notice periods:

> We're not on a lease at present. We just go week to week; if they want to terminate us they've got to give us I think 60 days and the same for us. When we did move in we were on a lease but that expired and we didn't re-sign, we just went week to week. … Yes, I'm happy with that because it doesn't lock us into anything if we want to move.

Sometimes, tenants had actively opted against longer leases offered by their landlord. They preferred a periodic tenancy. Annchi had been in the same property in a medium-rent area of Melbourne for 13 years:

> Yes, last time they offered me to renew a contract for two years, but because it's two years and, at that time, my son already finished high school and we are thinking about moving to a bigger place, so we said, "No". The agent said, "Are you sure? Because renewing the contract the price will be fixed", but I know in the law that is not really fixed, they can also still - they can still increase it, so I said, "Yes, I'm sure", but well, we are still here now.

In general, long-term renters were unenthusiastic about long-term leases under current regulation which permits regular rent increases. They also valued their ability to leave at short notice. Ashleigh (high-rent Melbourne) saw both the advantages and disadvantages of having a longer term lease under current rent setting rules:

> You know what, I really wish we had longer leases in Australia. Really, like five, maybe even ten years. Because one of the huge disadvantages in Australia is that every six months, twelve months, your rent goes up without fail.

Others saw longer term leases in more negative terms as inhibiting their ability to move if they wished, as in the case of, Nigel who was unemployed and living alone in an outer suburb of Sydney:

Nigel:	I had a six month lease and I'm still here. So the real estate they're all right by that.
Interviewer:	Would you prefer to have a longer lease or?
Nigel:	No, I'm happy the way it is now because whenever I'm ready to move out they can't do nothing about it. So yeah. All I have to do is give them four weeks' notice and I can go whenever I like.

Rodney (outer Sydney) thought that leases benefited the landlord and periodic tenancies benefited the tenant:

> Yeah, I used to think … that the lease is good for the tenant but it is the other way around. The lease is good for the landlord. It makes it easy cos if you stay for a certain time after the lease expired it is much harder [to be told to leave]. I think I looked it up. It was 92 days written notice or something like that.

In brief, there is no clear link between being on a fixed term lease or periodic tenancy and insecurity. Some tenants wanted a fixed term lease to have stronger legal security for a set period. Others valued their greater de facto security under a periodic tenancy arrangement because there was no formal review point at which rents would likely rise, and they were entitled to a longer notice period to move out if required. There was relatively little interest in longer term leases among long term renters, reflecting that this was a hypothetical question for almost all of them. Longer term leases made little sense if the same provisions continued to apply about notice to vacate for reasons such as the landlord wishing to sell the property and uncapped rent increases.

De facto Insecurity: Negotiating Relationships with Landlords and Agents

Long-term renters have, by our definition, been renting for at least 10 years. Some had moved during their time as a renter for reasons not of their choosing while others had lived in the same property for many years. Our interviews revealed two tenant strategies for minimizing the risk of a forced move: keeping under the radar by being a 'good' tenant who is not 'troublesome' and trying to find out the likelihood of the landlord selling the property which would mean that they would need to move out.

Keeping Under the Radar: Being a "Good Tenant" and "Not Troublesome"

Adhering to lease conditions such as paying the rent on time and looking after the property—being a "good tenant"—will likely improve chances of continuing a tenancy. Tenants also reported that they engaged in other practices as well to avoid being seen as "troublesome". These included not requesting maintenance works or complaining about landlord inaction to fix problems in case this prompted a tenancy termination. This strategy could be broadly described as "going under the radar".

To put some numbers around this, our survey asked 600 renters (short and longer term) whether they had decided not to pursue a complaint in the last 12 months about a problem, thinking that the rent would go up or the landlord might ask them to leave it they did. Nearly a fifth of respondents (18%) said that this was the case (22% among LTRs). Whilst not definitive, this suggests that keeping below the radar in this way is a strategy employed by a significant proportion of tenants who harbour anxiety about the possibility of a forced move. This was particularly commonly reported by households with dependent children and older tenants.

This strategy meant tenants trying to deal with maintenance problems themselves rather than bringing them to the attention of the agent or landlord. Maria and her partner in an inner Sydney suburb, tried to look after the property issues themselves to avoid attracting the landlord's attention.

> The corner of our bedroom there was mould growing because of the moisture in the wall because it is an old building and we just clean [it] ourselves and we don't tell them that that is a problem. We're just worried that if we say we have this issue they might say, "Okay, we want you to move out because we want to repaint the whole apartment", or "We want to make changes to the apartment", so we keep it quiet.

Ravi, a single man aged about 50 living an inner Melbourne suburb, relied on being a good tenant as a means of improving security. He had found what he considered a "gem of a place" that he wanted to keep. Part of his strategy was to keep regular property inspection transactions as short as possible:

> Because they come in here and they're like "Oh look, you obviously look after the place." They kind of walked in and went "Oh wow" and then "This is all good. Do you need anything?" and I'm like, "No". "No, everything's good. Okay, bye." ... Yeah, pay the rent on time, don't ask for anything, all good.

Not drawing attention to oneself was not just about the inside of a property. Kiera in her late 30s, living with her daughter in a middle suburb of Melbourne, was concerned about the impermanence of renting and feeling beholden to other people. She responded by keeping the front verge sufficiently neat so "that I won't draw attention to myself which will remind the real estate".

Many prided themselves on being "good tenants". For example, Fred and Winnie (outer Sydney) tried to keep the place as clean and tidy as possible which suited Winnie who said that she liked a very clean house.

Winnie: I don't like clutter, I don't like dirt that's why our real estates want to keep us because we've been with them since we came back from Orange. That is 15 years we've been with the same agent......

Fred: Not bragging but we have got what they call a triple A rating. So we can get a house anywhere we want. It is just affording it.

There was an awareness amongst tenants in low- rent areas about the consequences of asking for something to be done and getting on the radar of landlords and agents. Raelene was a single woman in her late 30s. She was acutely conscious that her property in outer Melbourne was someone else's family home and that tenants needed to be reliable to develop trust with a small-scale landlord:

> Yeah. I suppose if you're reliable before, and they trust you, in their family's house. There's not many good tenants around that don't trash the place.

On the other hand, Nirmal who lived with his wife and son in an outer suburb of Melbourne had used being a 'good tenant' as a negotiating tactic when notified of a rent increase they believed unfair. He researched median prices for rental properties in their area and presented this information to their property manager. This led to the rent increase being rescinded:

> I said, "Look, I'm a good tenant. I can get another property, but you won't get a good tenant like me." That was my straightforward answer, "and you're going to end up paying more money because as soon as I move out you're going to have to paint this whole house, fix all the doors, fix everything -" and I had a point.

In sum, a strategy employed by many of those interviewed was to keep under the radar as much as possible. This involved presenting themselves as a "good tenant" by paying the rent and having clean and tidy premises during an inspection and not asking for too much to be done for fear of the consequences of being seen as "troublesome" (see Power & Gillon, 2020). Trading off property condition against keeping rents from increasing was a means through which tenants in all housing market contexts tried to maximise their de facto security.

Developing Relationships with Landlords and Agents

In Sydney and Melbourne most tenancies are managed by real estate agents who mediate the relationship between landlord and tenant. In our survey of Sydney and Melbourne tenants, 87% rented through a real estate agent. Notwithstanding the important role of agents, one of the interesting ways in which long-term tenants and older tenants tried to work within the system of fixed term and periodic tenancies was to try to discover the landlord's identity to provide some basis for guessing their intentions on continuing to rent out the property. Landlord decisions to sell the property usually with vacant possession and, to a lesser extent, the landlord and/or their family moving back in, were the main risks to their tenancy.

Perhaps surprisingly, tenants felt more secure if the landlord owned more than one rental property. Danka was in her 30s and was in the fourth year of renting by herself in an inner Melbourne suburb. She had sent a letter to get her initial 12-month lease renewed but "nothing happened". She explained that:

> Usually I would feel a little bit uncomfortable about that, like I would have followed up and made sure that the lease was renewed but from what I can, have worked out from living here, all of these apartments are owned by one person and they just rent them out and they're all done through the same real estate agent. So as long as I'm paying my rent, I don't think they're going to kick me out …

Lenka who lived in an outer Melbourne suburb also knew about the landlord's plans for her property. Asked whether the landlord was thinking about selling the property, she replied:

> "Not in his lifetime", he said. He's got several investment properties and when he leaves us, he's basically done that for his children. He has four children. Obviously I don't know the agreements that they will have but he indicated to me at the time that it was unlikely. The only time that the properties may be sold is if his children decide to do that down the track and do the subdivisions, as is what's happening around here.

Chloe who lived with another adult in a sharer arrangement in an outer Sydney suburb, when asked about whether she was worried about security, said:

> Not really cos especially in this house because the same person owns all four so he hasn't bought this to live in at any time. He's bought this wholly as an investment, so to me that's more a security. If someone has bought the house and intend to live in it or they've lived in it then you worry. But if they bought it wholly as an investment and nothing else you are normally pretty secure as long as you do the right thing.

Many tenants were anxious to have some idea of the likelihood that the owner would either want to move in themselves, have their family move in, or sell the property—and to have advance warning if this was in prospect. This involved what they saw as an agreement with the landlord and/or managing agent which was built on trust. Frieda renting a property with four children in an outer Sydney put it like this:

> Yeah, it's just you know everything's done, everything that they've asked us to do, we've done. Or everything we've asked them to do, it has been done, so there's no you know like and no talk of or chatter about you know having to go or whatever … Cos normally you hear a little bit before that letter actually comes.

Raelene, who we met earlier in this chapter, had had direct contact with the owner of her rented property in Melbourne; on the basis of this she did not believe that the owner would sell. Most importantly, based on a conversation with the owner, she understood that the landlord would tell them if she changed her mind:

Interviewer: Do you feel that you feel safe that she is not going to want to sell this and then you're going to have to move again?

Raelene: No, she's not thinking of selling. She did say that if she was going to think about selling, that she would tell me.

Some tenants saw building a relationship with the managing agent as important to their security. Catherine, an older tenant living in Sydney, had a good relationship with her real estate agent. She was confident of being able to stay as long as she liked but also aware that selling the property is a decision of the landlord not the agent:

> I would like to be in something that we were renting permanently and know that you're there till you expire, but at the moment I feel as if we could be tossed out of the house or something, [although the agent] assures me we can stay here as long as we like. But you never know what's around the corner. They might have to sell the property some time for themselves because they have young families.

Despite trying to interpret the landlord's plans for their home, some tenants were concerned about the amount of knock-down-rebuild (redevelopment) activity in their area of Sydney or Melbourne. The high value of land where redevelopment at greater density was permitted could tempt the landlord to sell to a developer. For example, Danka (inner Melbourne) commented:

> I think that if you're in a rental that's always like a possibility. Like they could decide that they're going to pull this place down and build a high-rise here. But I don't think that's ever really worried me because I've got quite a big family so if something happened I'd always have somewhere to go.

Uncertainty about selling for redevelopment was also an issue in middle and outer suburbs as well. Kiera (middle suburb of Melbourne) put it like this:

> I mean it's never secure because it is someone else's place, but it is also frustrating because I know the system better than they seem to. …… Because the house in the street, I think I spoke to a person earlier this year, went for $1.5 million and you're like I wonder if suddenly the owner will decide now is a good time to sell or whatever because they're merrily pulling down all the old houses in the street.

In short, knowing something about the landlord and their situation was important to some tenants in moderating feelings of insecurity. Risks were considered lower where the landlord owned multiple properties. Of course, there was always a possibility of the landlord passing on and family members deciding to sell. The pressure of redevelopment in Sydney and Melbourne added to insecurity in that rising land values could tempt landlords to cash in on capital gains even where there were long-term tenants.

Perceptions of Insecurity

The research discussed earlier in the chapter suggests that there is variation in the ways in which people perceive housing insecurity despite apparently similar current housing situations. In the survey, renters were asked whether they felt that they would be able to live in their current dwelling for as long as they liked.

Perhaps surprisingly in view of their legal status, and notwithstanding the strategies that tenants used to try and achieve de facto security, three quarters of respondents were confident that they would not be faced with a forced move. There was some difference between short-term renters and LTRs with 9% of the former and 16% of the latter not feeling that they would be able to stay as long as they choose to. The main reasons cited were uncertainty about whether the landlord would continue to rent out the property and the affordability of the rent.

To unpack these responses further, we identified three common patterns among long-term and older tenants on this issue: insecurity is always at the back of your mind; constantly feeling insecure; and valuing the flexibility associated with being a tenant.

Insecurity "At the Back of My Mind"

The most common response that emerged from our interviews with long-term renters and older tenants was the sense of insecurity "at the back of my mind". This was mainly about the possibility that they would be asked to leave at short notice to allow for property sale, as discussed earlier in the chapter. Other possible forced move scenarios included a landlord wanting the property for themselves or their family or an unaffordable rent increase prompting the need to find somewhere cheaper.

Many tenants living in higher rent inner suburbs described such risks as something that they had had to learn to live with as long-term tenants. In different ways, they had resources (financial and support from family) to help them if this happened. Graham (inner-Sydney) described it like this:

> The security I suppose if you've always got that in the back of your mind that sort of impacts a little bit on your enjoyment, so I think that'd be the main thing.

Rebecca, living by herself in an inner Sydney suburb, pointed how out adapting to uncertainty in this way can still be shattered by a letter or a phone call:

> You know I'm conscious of the fact that I could be asked to leave at any time and when I got the call saying the valuer wanted to come through I panicked cos I thought okay they're going to sell and this is what's happened to me before, so that was my immediate reaction.

The valuer was sent by the real estate agent as the owner was looking to sell. Requesting access to her home for valuation purposes was the first time that she was aware of this. Liz also lived alone and had rented the same apartment in an inner

Sydney suburb for 15 years. Notwithstanding the length of her tenancy, she had at the back of her mind that the landlord might choose to sell:

> I mean, as I said, I've been lucky but I guess always in the back of my mind and this is I guess more for the disadvantage is that at some point the person who owns the property might want to sell it. I know people who have had to go through open houses you know like their places being on display and had to have the open house thing for weeks.

When asked whether she felt able to stay as long as she lived, Liz's reply indicated the financial resources that she had to deal with such a situation:

> Well I'd like to think so, but I'd be too scared to think about it too deeply. ... Like I mean obviously if the [owner] decided they would sell I would definitely put in an offer but financially I could afford to go and stay somewhere else or that might prompt me to buy something else. I have the security of enough money in the bank that wouldn't cause an issue or cause any problems.

Some of the older tenants took a similar view although many had considerably less resources than Liz. They had become familiar with rental insecurity. Raymond (older tenant, Sydney) put it this way:

> There's a stress factor, but it's not significant. The stress factor is that I occasionally think, "God, I wonder how long I can be here before somebody turfs me out", but ... I don't worry about it every day. I used to I must say when I first went from home owner to renter. I used to sweat over it a bit, but now I've been a renter for 14 years I don't think about it much.

Constantly Insecure

In contrast, some LTRs particularly in low and middle rent areas of Sydney and Melbourne, felt constantly insecure. Frieda, renting with her four children in an outer Sydney suburb was in this situation:

> It just made everything hard .... The kids didn't know from one day to the next whether they'd still be you know there or packing up again and going. I mean the first two they basically left their stuff in boxes and you know only their clothes were out and that was it. Where now they're like comfortable and everything is, their rooms' done the way they want their rooms done and yeah.

Michaela was in her late 50s having her adult daughter live with her temporarily in an outer Sydney suburb. She graphically described her perception of insecurity:

> You're constantly thinking, "Oh my god, you know what if they sell the house and then I've got to go? Where am I going to go? What am I going to do?" If you don't have money in the bank to help, to move on to another place like you know it's a matter of yeah, what's going to happen? And you do get anxious and like you say, you don't sleep and your mind's going constantly thinking about it, yeah.

Michaela went on to elaborate on the effects of constant insecurity despite renting her current home for 16 years. As she was on a Centrelink benefit she had the rent taken out of her benefit by direct debit. This left her $80 a fortnight for bills:

> You've always got that fear that you're not going to have a roof over your head at some stage. Yes, I've been here 16 years but you never know, the house can be sold and new owners say, "No we want you to go". You know what happens to you if someone comes along, like my situation my benefit pays all my rent. I have nothing to save and then they sell the house and the new owner says you have to go. You don't have money for a bond, for another premises or you know Housing Department can't help you because you're not, what they consider to be urgent.

Paul, introduced earlier in this chapter, also described the effect of constant insecurity:

> I have to be able and prepared to … move everything in a three month time-frame. … I do need to make sure that … I could call on the finances, get it all sorted, find a place, make that uproot change … I've done it a few times now, so I've got a much better handle on what it is that's needed to be done but again it's there. Just that little thing that sits in the back of your head. I couldn't - I mean I've travelled a few times but I can't really … I can't be away out of the country for extended periods of time because if the landlord did decide to give me 90 days and I'm out of the country for a month, then that would be a serious impact, so yeah.

Constant anxiety based on insecurity can have damaging effects on health and well-being. Natalie, an older renter in the Hawksbury area, an hour from Sydney, explained how she was affected very personally.

Natalie:	I became so aware of my insecurity that I lost the capacity to laugh, people have noticed the difference in me now that I was even three months ago.
Interviewer:	So sounds like you were depressed?
Natalie:	Yeah, I probably was but I didn't realise it because you know some of us can rise above it mostly. I probably if I had to go another year I just might have cracked up quite possible because you can get to that stage where what is it for. What is the point and when you reach a certain stage and age in your life, yes it does matter because what are your aspirations from the age of 79 onwards?

It is hard to overstate the way in which perceptions of constant insecurity affect the lives of some private renters. This is particularly accentuated for those who are on very low incomes and have few, if any, resources to draw on from family or friends and includes some older renters who are especially vulnerable. Some of these older renters had applied for social rental housing to improve their situation but as waiting list were long, the wait seemed interminable.

Flexibility as the Flip Side of Insecurity

Some private renters viewed the absence of long-term certainty associated with private renting in more positive terms. This may be an adaptive response in which some LTRs said that they valued the flexibility of renting in their current circumstances and current stage in life. For example, Amber lived with her partner and three children in an inner suburb of Sydney. She liked the flexibility of renting while she and her husband ran their own business. She expected to become a home owner in the future when able to extract money from the business.

Others choose to rent so that they can live in a suburb in which they could not afford to buy. For parents, this can be associated with prioritizing a location convenient for a preferred school. This was the case with Brooke, living with her partner, two young children and an au pair in an inner Sydney suburb:

> Yeah, but we choose to be renters because we choose to be in the suburb we're in so we choose the suburb for our children rather than the security of you know living in bricks and mortar. ... I'm going to work and I want to be able to get home from work within a reasonable amount of time. I also want the person who is looking after my children to be able to not have to be in a car driving them around. I think it is too unsafe. So they are the things that mean a lot to me more than ... knowing that this backyard is mine for the next whenever.

Among those expressing little concern about insecurity, some had come to terms with being a long-term renter. This type of security was often seemingly underpinned by financial resources and/or confidence in the knowledge of family support. Some had been in situations where they had been forced to rethink their priorities. This was true for Kitty who was in her early 70s and lived by herself in an inner suburb of Melbourne. Kitty had had cancer and been through gruelling treatment; this experience had caused her to rethink her priorities—and her life:

> So eventually I retired and I've done volunteer stuff that I've been interested in different areas, because they said, "You have to stop work, you can't go on working", and so that really probably is when I decided, "Well I'm not going to buy something. I'm going to enjoy my life". Because if I bought a house, I actually couldn't travel, even if I bought an apartment, because I'm not earning money to pay off the mortgage. And I do have enough money to buy quite a nice apartment, but I'd rather use the interest and the share money and stuff to travel, so that's my solution.

For the most part, renters who talked positively about flexibility and freedom were less home centred; at least at their current life stage and had more resources to draw on. They valued the ability to travel and have other types of experiences because they were not tied to a mortgage. This is perhaps encapsulated by Anne and her partner who were both working full-time but had other priorities at this stage in their life:

> Yeah, so this is like you have control of your life with finances. You can invest in things that are not necessarily just a house. You can invest in things that are part of what you see as other areas of life–and it sounds like travel and experiences such as food and entertainment is very important isn't it?

In sum, perceptions of insecurity among private renters varied considerably, in what is becoming an increasingly diverse population. Some had the financial resources and social connections if they had to move whilst, most commonly, long term renters put insecurity to the back of their minds as they got on with their daily lives. A group of private renters, including some older renters, were constantly worried about the insecurity of their position to the extent that it affected their health and wellbeing.

Control and Choice

Underlying experiences of de facto insecurity and perceived insecurity are some important issues about control and choice. The research literature points to a lack of control underlying the psycho-social dimensions of housing insecurity such as lack of autonomy (Hulse & Saugeres, 2008) and is ambivalent on the issue of choice, since no-one has unconstrained choice of living arrangements and often different priorities must be balanced, or traded off, against each other.

Control

Tenant interviewees in all housing market contexts talked in depth about control—over their housing and their lives. Some expressed strong concern about lack of, of loss of, control over their lives. For example, Louise (inner Sydney) was concerned about a loss of control over her life:

> Insecurity of tenure and unpredictability that factor the unpredictability for the future and then the loss of control over your life the way you would like your life to be going are the key factors. That make it [long term renting] very disadvantageous.

She was also concerned about the effects of insecurity and lack of control on her teenage son: "I hate … the thought that my son is being made to feel insecure in some way".

Gina (outer suburb of Sydney) was also concerned about the impact of insecurity on her young daughter:

> Not being able to stay in [a rental property], not being able to create a family home where you are comfortable, you know that you're going to stay there you know that you're not going to have to. … the main thing is for the children not for us – like growing up you'd like to be able to have them in one home you know especially the little one, you know. She doesn't understand that we rent. She doesn't understand like the concept of renting. She thinks it's her house and she sees the sign going up and she's like what. She just asks a million questions. What's going on?

Brooke (inner Sydney) although appearing to be very well-resourced, also expressed concern about lack of control, particularly having a young baby to care for:

> Look, I don't feel like I'm in control. Like the real estate will ring up and say, I need to come and do x, y and z and tell you when she's coming and not necessarily give a damn. They put the place on the market and I had a six week old baby, cleaning twice a week so that they could present it and I bothered to clean like I didn't have to. Plenty of the other tenants didn't, but we had to be out of the place twice a week you know [the real estate agent] did have the decency to [ask] what's the best time of day to do that.

Not everyone felt that this lack of control associated with private renting had a profound effect on their life. For example, Sarah who lived with her husband and four children in an inner Melbourne suburb had a different approach to the link between security and control:

> Well, I do have control over my life, yeah. And actually, I think not long ago my sister said, "What about if they kick you out?" ... And my response is, "Well, then I'll work it out." We'll just ... I'm not worried about it.

For others, a sense of control was more nuanced. For example, Lenka had lived in the same property in outer Melbourne for 16 years:

> I know that I'm always going to be at the mercy of the owners and the agents, so I can't control what they decide. Otherwise, I feel like I have complete control over what happens on the property while I'm here. Because I do have that freedom to treat it as my own, to treat it like home. But it's still always I think going to be in the back of your mind, what if?

Choice

An interesting, and perhaps unexpected theme in the interviews was that some private renters considered that indebted home owners did not have much better security than private renters and that paying off a mortgage limited home owners' lives compared to renters. This view was articulated across different types of households and different housing market contexts.

Ravi aged 50 (inner Melbourne) did not see much difference between renting and purchasing:

> Look, I think if you're paying rent or you're paying mortgages, intrinsically it's a very similar amount of money. You know, it's a matter of financial freedom or having surplus cash. To me, it was always about being able to work and live in reasonably close proximity to each other.

Nirmal (outer Melbourne) talked about people paying off their mortgages who were in a bad situation.

> [They] made those decisions at the wrong point of time and now they've ended up paying a lot more what they're doing now and as a result it's causing a bit of a mental stress in terms of, I've got the mortgage next month, I've got to pay this off, and they've compromised with their living standards. At this point in time we don't have to compromise with living standards. We can eat whatever we want, and we can save as well. We've been able to save a fair bit of money staying in this house.

Some of those interviewed considered that they were better off renting than having a huge mortgage in terms of lifestyle. Sophie who was in her mid 30s and living with her partner and baby in a middle suburb of Sydney, put it this way:

> the area where we want to live and have sort of more of the lifestyle we want to have is more important to us than whether we own our own home or not. Whereas I know a lot of people some people who I work with and other people I know their priority is own their own home, beyond everything else. They will eat two-minute noodles and not go anywhere and drive a 20-year-old car because they have to own their own home whereas that's not the number one priority in my life.

Buying houses with a large mortgage that was difficult to repay was seen by some renters as being conformist without thinking through the consequences. Rodney put it this way:

> And it has become the Stepford way, conform to society. All the people slaving away to own a house. All they do is have a little dinner parties in each other's house and all they can afford is cheap bottles of wine and some chicken kievs and the kids running around and destroy the place they're working so hard to [afford] … It just seems it is social conformity that I don't think I fit into either.

Conclusion

Australia's private renters have relatively little legal security but it is clear that landlord-tenant relationships, often mediated by real estate agents, are negotiated through social practices. Beyond "being a good tenant" by paying the landlord on time and looking after the place, renters often attempt to reduce the risk of rent increases and tenancy termination by striving to remain below the radar of landlords and agents. Avoiding acquiring a "troublesome tenant" reputation can involve keeping quiet about necessary repairs or replacement items in case the rent goes up as a result and the tenant has to leave. This can be seen as a manifestation of a power imbalance between landlords and tenants since many of those interviewed pointed to work that they thought needed to be done on their property.

Tenants also try to manage their legal insecurity by endeavouring to find out about the landlord's situation as a basis for better guessing their possible future plans for the property. They feel more secure when their landlord owns several properties as they are then unlikely to want to move themselves or their families back in, requiring the tenant to vacate. Some private renters see this as a relationship of trust, sometimes via the agent, but they recognise that unexpected events affecting the landlord such as illness or death may still lead to property sale and a consequential need to depart at relatively short notice. While these factors are quite specific and personal, there is also a more general and growing concern about rising land values which might prompt property redevelopment, affecting the de facto security of long-term and older tenants.

The way that insecurity is perceived, and its effect on tenants' lives varies according to factors such as age, responsibility for children and the financial and non-financial resources that tenants have to back them up. There are also quite significant individual differences in how tenants respond to insecurities with some being constantly worried to the extent that their health is affected while others appear unconcerned and value the flexibility that renting can provide in a periodic tenancy scenario. By far the most common response among tenants is that insecurity is "at the back of the mind"; an omnipresent concern but one which might not be at the forefront of daily concerns. The chapter has shown that tenants have diverse views on the extent of choice and control that they are able to exercise in their lives and the contribution of housing insecurity to the ways in which they want to live their lives.

Housing insecurity can also explode unexpectedly in the face of society-wide events as the COVID-19 pandemic of 2020–21 has shown. Events of this, and lesser magnitude, will heighten housing insecurity and reduce a sense of control. Those with higher levels of financial security, personal support and social connectedness will certainly be better able to weather these storms. The COVID pandemic of 2020–21 has highlighted that Australian governments have struggled to find and reach agreement on measures to address extreme housing insecurity experienced by private tenants as a consequence of losing their jobs. This puts the spotlight on which types of actions might best deal with housing insecurity for private renters in such extreme circumstances: regulatory change, income support measures, targeted rental support, moratoria on evictions, tax reductions for landlords, and/or landlord-tenant negotiation on rent levels. We reflect on the future of the private rental sector in the post COVID-19 era in the next, and concluding, chapter.

References

ABS. (2019). *Household income and wealth, Australia, 2017–18* (Cat. no. 6523.0). Canberra, ACT: Australian Bureau of Statistics.

Australian Bureau of Statistics (ABS). (2013). *Counts of Australian businesses, including entries and exits, June 2009 to June 2013* (Cat. No. 8165.0). Canberra, ACT: Australian Bureau of Statistics.

Australian Taxation Office (ATO). (2018). *Taxation statistics 2015–16*. Canberra, ACT: Australian Taxation Office. https://www.ato.gov.au/About-ATO/Research-and-statistics/In-detail/Taxation-statistics/Taxation-statistics-2015-16/?page=6#Individuals_detailed_tables.

Blunden, H., & Martin, C. (2004). *Leaking roofs: Australian tenancy law: A report by the National Association of Tenants Organisations*. Sydney, NSW: Tenants Union of NSW.

Campbell, I., & Burgess, J. (2018). Patchy progress? Two decades of research on precariousness and precarious work in Australia. *Labour & Industry, 28*(1), 48–67.

Dupuis, A., & Thorns, D. (1998). Home, home ownership and the search for ontological security. *Sociological Review, 46*(1), 24–47.

Fitzpatrick, S., & Pawson, H. (2014). Ending security of tenure for social renters: Transitioning to 'ambulance service' social housing? *Housing Studies, 29*(5), 597–615.

Fitzpatrick, S., & Watts, B. (2017). Competing visions: Security of tenure and the welfarisation of English social housing. *Housing Studies, 32*(8), 1021–1038.

Hiscock, R., Kearns, A., Macintyre, S., & Ellaway, A. (2001). Ontological security and psycho-social benefits from the home: Qualitative evidence on issues of tenure. *Housing, Theory and Society, 18*(10), 50–66.

Hulse, K., Martin, C., James, A. 4 Stone, W. (2018a). *Private rental in transition: Institutional change, technology and innovation in Australia*, No. 296. Melbourne, VIC: AHURI. https://doi.org/10.18408/ahuri-5112101.

Hulse, K., & Milligan, V. (2014). Secure occupancy: A new framework for analysing security in rental housing. *Housing Studies, 29*(5), 638–656. https://doi.org/10.1080/02673037.2013.873116.

Hulse, K., Milligan, V. & Easthope, H. (2011). *Secure occupancy in rental housing: Conceptual foundations and comparative perspectives*, No. 170. Melbourne, VIC: AHURI.

Hulse, K., Morris, A., & Pawson, H. (2019a). Private renting in a home ownership society: Disaster, diversity or deviance? *Housing Theory and Society, 36*(2), 167–188. https://doi.org/10.1080/14036096.2018.1467964.

Hulse, K., Parkinson, S. & Martin, C. (2018b). *Inquiry into the future of the private rental sector*, No. 303. Melbourne, VIC: AHURI. https://doi.org/10.18408/ahuri-5112001.

Hulse, K., Reynolds, M., Nygaard, C., Parkinson, S. & Yates, J. (2019b). *The supply of affordable private rental housing in Australian cities: Short-term and longer-term changes*, No. 323. Melbourne, VIC: AHURI. https://doi.org/10.18408/ahuri5120101.

Hulse, K., & Saugeres, L. (2008). *Housing insecurity and precarious living in Australian rental housing*, No. 124. Melbourne, VIC: Australian Housing and Urban Research Institute (AHURI).

Kearns, A., Hiscock, R., Ellaway, A., & Macintyre, S. (2000). "Beyond four walls": The psychosocial benefits of home: Evidence from west central Scotland. *Housing Studies, 15*(3), 387–410.

Leopold, J., Cunningham, M., Posey, L. & Manuel, T. (2016). *Improving measures of housing insecurity: A path forward*. Washington, DC: The Urban Institute. https://www.urban.org/sites/default/files/publication/101608/improving_measures_of_housing_insecurity.pdf.

Martin, C., Hulse, K. & Pawson, H. (2018). *The changing institutions of private rental housing: An international review*, No. 292. Melbourne, VIC: AHURI. https://doi.org/10.18408/ahuri-7112201.

Minnery, J., Adkins, B., Grimbeek, P. Summerville, J., Mead, E. & Guthrie, D. (2003). *Tenure security and its impact on private renters in Queensland*, No. 27. Melbourne, VIC: AHURI.

Morris, A. (2016). *The Australian dream: Housing experiences of older Australians*. Melbourne, VIC: CSIRO Publishing.

Morris, A. (2018). Housing tenure and the health of older Australians dependent on the age pension for their income. *Housing Studies, 33*(1), 77–95.

Morris, A., Hulse, K., & Pawson, H. (2017). Long-term private renters: Perceptions of security and insecurity. *Journal of Sociology, 53*(3), 653–669.

National Association of Tenant Organisations (NATO), Carr & Tennant. (2010). *A better lease on life: Improving Australian tenancy law*. Canberra, ACT: National Shelter.

Pawson, H., Hulse, K., & Morris, A. (2017). Interpreting the rise of long-term private renting in a liberal welfare regime context. *Housing Studies, 32*(8), 1062–1084. https://doi.org/10.1080/02673037.2017.1301400.

Power, E. (2017). Renting with pets: A pathway to housing insecurity? *Housing Studies, 32*(3), 336–360.

Power, E. R., & Gillon, C. (2020). Performing the 'good tenant'. *Housing Studies*. https://doi.org/10.1080/02673037.2020.1813260.

Soatia, A., Munro, M. & McKee, K. (2020). *Private renters' housing experiences in lightly regulated markets*. Glasgow: UK Collaborative Centre for Housing Evidence. https://housingevidence.ac.uk/wp-content/uploads/2020/04/200429_PRS_evidence_review_final.pdf.

Webb, E. (2018). Housing an ageing Australia: The ideal of security of tenure and the undermining effect of elder abuse. *Macquarie Law Journal, 18*, 57–78.

Chapter 8
Conclusions: Living with Uncertainty

Abstract This chapter summarises our main arguments and findings and reflects on the possible impacts of the Covid-19 pandemic on the private rental sector. We argue that the high cost of housing relative to incomes and the near stagnation in the building of social housing, has meant that for an increasing proportion of Australians private renting is their only option. Despite its ever-increasing importance, the sector remains lightly regulated. This is reflected most clearly in the capacity of landlords in most Australian states to terminate a tenancy without having to give a reason. A key contribution of the book is the in-depth exploration of tenants' experiences and perspectives on private renting. The coverage of rental situations across low, medium and high-rent areas and on Age Pension-reliant tenants has highlighted the extreme diversity of the private renting experience. For middle and high income earners, private renting is often viewed favourably at least in the short-medium term. However, for low-income private renters, being a private renter can be extremely challenging due to the cost of the accommodation relative to income and the perpetual insecurity. The loss of employment and income related to the pandemic in areas such as hospitality and tourism has certainly accentuated the difficulties of many low-income renters. We conclude that a fundamental shift in the way housing is viewed is required if Australia's housing system is to become more equitable and affordable. Rather than the maxim that market forces will provide, and people need to find their own way, affordable and secure housing must be reconceptualised as a human right.

Private Renting: Growth, Institutional Settings and Tenant Experiences

In the era of reconstruction after WW2, Australia became a nation of home owners and private renting entered a steep decline, reaching its lowest point in the mid-1960s. For the next two decades, private renting was mainly a transitional sector for young people and immigrants prior to home ownership. From the mid-1980s, however, a slow revival began, accelerating in the 2000s and 27% of households are now private renters. The sector's transitional role has been weakening as a large proportion of

A. Morris et al., *The Private Rental Sector in Australia*,
https://doi.org/10.1007/978-981-33-6672-5_8

renters are no longer able to exit into home ownership and there are more renters at midlife and post-retirement age.

We argue that the high cost of housing relative to incomes, especially in Sydney and Melbourne, the declining availability of social housing and a labour market characterised by high rates of underemployment and low and insecure wages, means that for an ever-increasing proportion of Australians, the PRS is their only housing option. Especially for young adults, home ownership is unattainable in the short-to-medium term, if ever. Between 1986 and 2016, the home ownership rate among 25–34 year-olds fell from 55.6 to 44.6% and among 34–44 year-olds from 73.2 to 62.2% (Burke et al., 2020, p. 32). The high levels of unemployment and under-employment due to the COVID-19 pandemic is likely to accentuate this trend.

PRS growth has been facilitated by the financialisation of housing—the increasing dominance of financial actors, markets and practices (Aalbers, 2016)—such that residential property is increasingly viewed as an investment and commodity rather than a place to live. A policy regime endorsed by successive Australian governments has encouraged the view that small-scale landlordism is highly desirable as a means of self-provisioning for older age as well as providing a much needed boost to the rental supply (Hulse et al., 2020). It has contributed to "mum and dad" landlord dominance; an estimated 2.2 million people, one in every seven Australian households now owns an "investment property".

A long-standing theme of academic analysis has been the inadequacies and inconsistencies of state legislation on residential tenancies. Whilst there have been improvements since state landlord-tenant legislation was described as "a scandal" at the time of the 1970s Poverty Inquiry (Bradbrook, 1975), some of the most important recommendations for change remain to be adopted. In almost all of Australia, once the written tenancy agreement ends, a landlord can terminate the contract with no reasons required. The capacity for no grounds termination severely weakens tenants' ability to challenge inadequate maintenance or unjustified rent increases. Further, when it comes to the imposition of higher rents, the onus remains on tenants to dispute the reasonableness thereof, rather than for landlords to demonstrate their legitimacy (NATO et al., 2010).

A key contribution of the book is the in-depth exploration of tenants' experiences and perspectives on private renting in Australia's two biggest cities. The coverage of rental situations across low, medium and high-rent areas is distinctive, as is the emphasis on long-term renters in a variety of circumstances and on Age Pension-reliant tenants. This approach has highlighted the extreme diversity of the private renting experience. Although all tenants have similar *de jure* (legal) situations, our research highlights their highly varied capacity to enjoy a decent life in this housing situation. As discussed in Chapter 1, the association between private renting and poverty has been well-recognised for almost a hundred years. However, the last few decades have also seen an increase in middle and higher-income households unable to afford home ownership in a chosen area, thanks in part to the steepened price gradient between higher priced inner-city housing and lower prices on the outskirts of cities and in regional areas. A professional employed couple renting in an amenity rich inner-city area, will likely have a very different residential experience and concerns to a single parent or an Age Pension-reliant tenant in an outer area. We show that the variations operate at every stage of the private renter experience—the decision to rent, the search for a tenancy, the capacity to create a home, the ability to afford the rent, perceptions of [in]security and future housing plans.

Some of our interviewees had been previously in a comfortable housing position, but adverse life events such as marital dissolution or separation or the onset of chronic illness or disability had a shattering impact on their housing situation and prospects. When occurring in middle age, a common outcome is one or both parties being pushed out of home ownership and into private rental. Enforced reliance on the PRS can be extremely difficult for people in this situation. For Age Pension recipients whose circumstances were unlikely to improve, the only possible alternative was a social housing tenancy with better security and lower rent. However, invariably they faced long years on the waiting list. As also illustrated from our interviews, for younger people separation or divorce can have a profound impact on home ownership prospects. For many, plans to purchase a home had been crushed and they now faced long-term or even lifelong tenant status.

A few of our interviewees, mainly living in the inner-city high-rent areas, had actively chosen to rent. They enjoyed the associated flexibility and the amenities in inner-city areas, including access to good quality government schools. They flinched at the thought of being "tied down" by a mortgage. Some had the capacity to buy a property, although perhaps not in their current neighbourhood. Others already owned a property elsewhere which they chose to rent out rather than occupy themselves.

The varying capacity to find and access a rental property is another highly differentiated feature across the private tenant population. Low-income renters, more especially those reliant on government benefits, often face extreme difficulty finding a suitable property and securing a tenancy offer in the normally highly competitive rental markets of Sydney and Melbourne. This can be a traumatic experience. Interviewees recounted submitting dozens of applications and being knocked back time after time. Some had reached a point where they feared that homelessness could result.

Nevertheless, once tenants had accessed a rental property, they generally found it possible to create a sense of home, despite enjoying only limited legal security. Only one in twenty respondents in our Sydney/Melbourne survey said that they did not feel at home "at all". The condition of the dwelling was an important factor. A reassuring finding was that eight in ten respondents agreed that their rental property was in good condition. Again, however, this was far less likely to be true for tenants reliant on government benefits; they were more often forced to accept a low-rent but rundown property.

A central factor determining a tenant's capacity to feel at home was their relationship with the landlord or agent. In situations where tenants felt secure, were treated respectfully, had maintenance issues promptly addressed and enjoyed the freedom to personalise their dwelling, it was likely that they would feel "at home". Interviewees in low-rent areas—typically low-income workers or benefit-reliant tenants—often reported enduring serious property issues but were reluctant to "make a fuss". They feared that pressing for problems to be fixed could provoke a rent increase or, at worst, trigger a request to vacate.

The association between private renting and poverty has been the subject of research and inquiries for many decades. The face of poverty in Australia has moved from private renters living in sub-standard and crowded cottages in inner-city areas in the early twentieth century to the more dispersed poverty of low-income private renters on city fringes where the most affordable rentals—and lower levels of transport, facilities and amenities—are now found. Tenants on low incomes, particularly government benefits, recounted their daily battles to purchase basic necessities. Any unexpected expense was a major blow. Many tenants in low-paid work were also battling with everyday expenses. Shockingly, our survey indicated that 15% of respondents in low-rent areas said that they had had to forego meals in the last year, whereas this was true for only 4% of respondents in medium and high rent areas—and 3% of households nationally (ABS, 2013).

With respect to insecurity there is considerable variation in tenants' de facto experiences of insecurity and in their perceptions. For many tenants in high and medium-rent areas, the legal insecurity intrinsic to the PRS is of relatively little concern and, for some, the low commitment required, and ease of exiting housing, is viewed as a positive advantage. The most common pattern was that insecurity was "at the back of mind". However, many low-income interviewees lived with a constant sense of insecurity. As highlighted by our evidence, constant anxiety about the risk of a forced move can be profoundly psychologically debilitating.

Back to the Future?

There are two possible scenarios for the sector's future trajectory: one is a continuation of trends to date in the twenty-first Century and the second is a paradigm shift in response to the COVID-19 pandemic. We briefly explore each possibility.

Continued Growth of Private Renting and More of the Same?

A continuation of recent trends (Hulse et al., 2019) will see an ongoing increase in private renting at about twice the rate of overall household growth. Tenants will become a larger and increasingly diverse group in terms of household incomes, age profile and stage in the life cycle and we will see more longer term renters and a prospect of lifelong renting for more households. This will present challenges for policies related to ageing, including retirement incomes, predicated on most people owning their home outright by the time they retire from the workforce (Yates & Bradbury, 2010). Rental markets will become yet more spatially differentiated with the lowest income renters increasingly segregated into outer suburban disadvantaged areas. There will be more small-scale landlords buying and selling their properties for capital gain, resulting in a churn in properties and more insecure tenancies. Incremental changes to residential tenancies legislation will continue, in which measures that benefit tenants are "balanced" against measures that benefit landlords and legal insecurity will likely persist.

This scenario will intensify social inequality (Coates & Chivers, 2019) between younger and older generations and between people living in different rental markets. Increasingly an individual's class origins will ultimately determine their housing status (Adkins et al., 2019). Children of parents who are renters will find it exceptionally difficult to access home ownership creating what has been called "The Renting Class" (Wiesel, 2016).

The COVID-19 Pandemic and Beyond

In the first few months of the pandemic in Australia, as elsewhere, the number of people unemployed, under-employed or no longer in the labour force rocketed (ABS, 2020). Government had to reimagine assistance to those paying off a mortgage and renters affected by job loss or reduced income. Tenants were particularly hard-hit (Baker et al., 2020; Morris et al., 2020). A survey of 15,000 renters conducted in July and August 2020 concluded,

> Large numbers of renting households have been thrown into precarious employment, or even unemployment, with many now finding it difficult to make housing payments. Tenure insecurity has become a pressing risk for many renters. (Baker et al., 2020, p. 2)

To counter the spectre of mass ejection from private rental, short-term eviction moratoria were installed by state governments, with landlords asked to consider rent reductions for tenants no longer able to afford existing rates. The moratoria on evictions came to an end at the end of March 2021. What has become apparent is that vacancy rates have increased, probably mainly due to younger people returning to the family home and the decline in international students. Consequently asking rents have been falling in Melbourne and Sydney, particularly for apartments, as landlords struggle to find tenants (Fitzsimmons, 2020; Heagney, 2020).

The pandemic may have long-term impacts for the PRS. These are likely to include disinvestment in rental properties by some landlords who need to recoup their equity and repay loans. The impacts on tenants will vary. Those who have managed to retain jobs will likely benefit from lower rents at least in the short-medium term. For tenants not in paid work, or underemployed, their situation will continue to be very difficult.

The Way Forward

Our research suggests that a far-reaching shift in the way housing is viewed is required if Australia's housing system is to progress along a more equitable and affordable path. Living with uncertainty can have pernicious effects on people's lives. Rather than the maxim that market forces will provide, and people need to find their own way, affordable and secure housing must be reconceptualised as a human right. This shift will necessitate significant government intervention. In the short-term, it will call for a redrafting of the legal framework around tenant-landlord relations, so as to increase the security and enhance the power of tenants. No grounds evictions need to be outlawed and longer notice periods for prescribed cause terminations introduced, particularly for longer term tenants. Our research suggests that tenants are concerned about the short notice period if landlords sell the property or decide to move in themselves or house family members. There needs to be a mechanism to cap the size of rent increases as occurs in countries like Germany discussed in Chapter 2. In cities with expensive rental markets, RA needs to be bolstered to take account of the high median rents.

A key requirement is policies to counter housing financialisation. The present tax regime, the real estate industry celebration of rising house prices and the typically uncritical media reportage of that perspective, have reshaped the way housing is viewed. Instead of housing being regarded primarily as a means to acquire secure and comfortable shelter, it is presented and seen by an increasing proportion of the population as an investment and a sure-fire way to accumulate wealth (Blunden, 2016; Martin, 2018). The resulting encouragement of property speculation is pernicious, since this further boosts house price inflation. This in turn shuts out a large proportion of potential home buyers and ensures their long-term PRS dependence (Morris, 2019; Pawson et al., 2017). The landlord investor tax reforms that could help to correct this situation have been widely rehearsed (Johnstone, 2010; Daley et al., 2016; Pawson et al., 2020).

A key finding of our study is that tenants reliant on government benefits or on very low wages are often profoundly insecure. For these households, private renting exacerbates problems of income poverty. Their minimal income means that they are extremely constrained with respect to the location and condition of their rental property and their capacity to withstand any rent increase. Their situation often evokes considerable anxiety and stress. That tenants reliant on social security are usually in a highly precarious situation is not surprising. A comparison of social security payments and poverty lines using 2015–2016 data concluded that even using the conservative poverty line, 50% of median income measure, all the payments were below the poverty line (Davidson et al., 2018). If the 60% of median income is used as the poverty line, the gap becomes considerable. In 2014, Australia was "the sixth lowest spender [on social security] of 35 OECD countries, spending slightly more than Turkey and slightly less than Israel …" (Whiteford, 2017, p. 21).

Older private renters were particularly stressed by their situation and anxious about a rent increase forcing them to move (see Morris, 2016). Although the adequacy of the Age Pension is premised on low housing costs, current trends suggest that the proportion of older Australians dependent on the PRS will expand substantially in the coming decades due to the increasing inability of low-income individuals and families to access home ownership. Grattan Institute projections anticipate that the proportion of older Australians in home ownership will drop from 76% at present to 57% by 2056 (Coates & Chen, 2019). Retirement income policies need to make sufficient provision for private rental costs rather than assuming outright home ownership in older age.

There will always be a sizeable section of the citizenry able to participate only marginally—if at all—in the mainstream economy. Rather than allowing this part of the population to suffer unduly (with high housing costs being a primary contributor), government needs to create an infrastructure of care; adequate social security benefits and an increased supply of affordable and adequate housing would be a key components of this infrastructure. In an increasingly uncertain world, this approach would improve the lives of those who suffer most in living with uncertainty.

References

Aalbers, M. B. (2016). *The financialization of housing: A political economy approach*. New York: Routledge.

ABS (Australian Bureau of Statistics). (2013). *4670.0—Household energy consumption survey*. Australia: Summary of Results, 2012; Table 25. https://www.abs.gov.au/AUSSTATS/abs@.nsf/DetailsPage/4670.02012?OpenDocument.

ABS (Australian Bureau of Statistics). (2019a). *6202.0 labour force, Australia, May 2020, media release, 18 June*. Canberra: ABS. https://www.abs.gov.au/ausstats/abs%40.nsf/mediareleasesbyCatalogue/F00771E26218DFB1CA258479001AAD2E.

ABS (Australian Bureau of Statistics). (2019b). *6202.0 labour force, Australia, Sep 2019*. Canberra: ABS.

ABS (Australian Bureau of Statistics). (2020, December). *Labour force Australia*. Table 1. https://www.abs.gov.au/statistics/labour/employment-and-unemployment/labour-force-australia/dec-2020.

Adkins, L., Cooper, M., & Konings, M. (2019). Class in the 21st century: Asset inflation and the new logic of inequality. *Environment and Planning A: Economy and Space*. https://doi.org/10.1177/0308518X19873673.

Baker, E., Bentley, R., Beer, A., & Daniel, L. (2020). *Renting in the time of COVID 19: Understanding the impacts*. AHURI Final Report No. 340, Australian Housing and Urban Research Institute Limited, Melbourne. https://www.ahuri.edu.au/research/final-reports/340; https://doi.org/10.18408/ahuri3125401.

Blunden, H. (2016). Discourses around negative gearing of investment properties in Australia. *Housing Studies, 31*(3), 340–357.

Bradbrook, A. J. (1975). *Poverty and the residential landlord-tenant relationship*. Canberra: Australian Government Publishing Service.

Burke, T., Nygaard, C., & Ralson, L. (2020). *Australian home ownership: Past reflections, future directions, AHURI final report 328*. Melbourne: Australian Housing and Urban Research Institute.

Coates, B., & Chen, T. (2019, April 12). Fewer retires will own their home in future, and that has big implications for policy. *The Conversation*. https://theconversation.com/retiree-home-ownership-is-about-to-plummet-soon-little-more-than-half-will-own-where-they-live-115255.

Coates, B., & Chivers, C. (2019, September 19). Rising inequality in Australia isn't about incomes: It's almost all about housing. *The Conversation.*

Daley, J., Wood, D., & Parsonage, H. (2016). *Hot property negative gearing and capital gains tax reform.* Melbourne: Grattan Institute.

Davidson, P., Saunders, P., Bradbury, B., & Wong, M. (2018). *Poverty in Australia, 2018.* Sydney: ACOSS/UNSW Poverty and Inequality Partnership report No 2. Sydney: ACOSS.

Duke, J. (2021, March 29). House prices were expected to fall, now they're tipped for a record rise. What's going on? *The Sydney Morning Herald.* https://www.smh.com.au/politics/federal/house-prices-were-expected-to-fall-now-they-re-tipped-for-a-record-rise-what-s-going-on-20210.

Elmas, M. (2021, April 15). Soaring rents add insult to injury in housing affordability crisis. *The New Daily.* https://thenewdaily.com.au/finance/finance-news/2021/04/15/rents-housing-affordability/.

Fitzsimmons, C. (2020, May 24). 'A very good time to upgrade': Tenant bag bargains as landlords drop rents. *Sydney Morning Herald.*

Heagney, M. (2020, July 8). Melbourne apartment rents fall for the first time in 15 years as COVID-19 hits the market. *Domain.* https://www.domain.com.au/news/melbourne-apartment-rents-fall-for-the-first-time-in-15-years-as-covid-19-hits-the-market-967505/.

Hulse, K., Reynolds, M., & Martin, C. (2020). The everyman archetype: Discursive reframing of private landlords in the financialization of rental housing. *Housing Studies, 35*(6), 981–1003. https://doi.org/10.1080/02673037.2019.1644297.

Hulse, K., Reynolds, M., Nygaard, C., Parkinson, S., & Yates, J. (2019). *The supply of affordable private rental housing in Australian cities: Short-term and longer-term changes*, AHURI Final Report 323. Melbourne: Australian Housing and Urban Research Institute.

Johnston, C. (2010). *Henry on housing: The Australia's future tax system reports; Shelter NSW Memo.* Sydney: Shelter NSW. http://pandora.nla.gov.au/pan/126448/20110411-1517/www.sheltersw.org.au/docs/mem1009comment-henryreview.pdf. Accessed 16 July 2019.

Martin, C. (2018). Clever Odysseus: Narratives and strategies of rental property investor subjectivity in Australia. *Housing Studies, 33*(7), 1060–1084.

Morris, A. (2016). *The Australian dream: Housing experiences of older Australians.* Melbourne: CSIRO Publishing.

Morris, A. (2019). An impossible task? Neoliberalism, the financialisation of housing and the City of Sydney's endeavours to address its housing affordability crisis. *International Journal of Housing Policy.* https://doi.org/10.1080/19491247.2019.1688634.

Morris, A., Hastings, C., Wilson, S., Mitchell, E., & Ramia, G. (2020). *The experience of international students before and during COVID-19: Housing, work, study and well-being.* Sydney: Institute for Public Policy and Governance, University of Technology Sydney. https://internationalstudentsandhousing.files.wordpress.com/2020/08/international-students-and-housing-survey-report-final-no-logos-5-aug-2020.pdf.

NATO, Carr, & Tennant. (2010). *A better lease on life: Improving Australian tenancy law.* Canberra: National Shelter.

Pawson, H., Hulse, K., & Morris, A. (2017). Interpreting the rise of long-term renting in a liberal welfare regime context. *Housing Studies, 32*(8), 1062–1084.

Pawson, H., Milligan, V., & Yates, J. (2020). *Housing policy in Australia: A case for system reform.* Singapore: Palgrave.

Pawson, H., Martin, C., Sisson, A., Thompson, S., Fitzpatrick, S., & Marsh, A. (2021). COVID-19: Rental housing and homelessness impacts—An initial analysis. ACOSS/UNSW Poverty and Inequality Partnership Report No. 7, Sydney. https://bit.ly/3p2er65.

Provisional University. (2016, February 1). *Vulture landlords: An in depth interview with Desiree Fields.* https://provisionaluniversity.wordpress.com/2016/02/01/vulture-landlords-an-in-depth-interview-with-desiree-fields/.

Razaghi, T. (2021, April 16). Byron rents now pricier than most of Sydney. *The Sydney Morning Herald.* https://www.domain.com.au/news/calls-for-rent-control-as-regional-town-tenants-experience-double-digit-jump-in-rents-1044768.

Whiteford, P. (2017, July). *Social security and welfare spending in Australia: Assessing long-term trends, TTPI—Policy Brief*. Canberra: Australian National University. https://taxpolicy.crawford.anu.edu.au/sites/default/files/uploads/taxstudies_crawford_anu_edu_au/2018-12/combined_pdf_whiteford_trends_in_soc_sec_spending_2017.pdf.

Wiesel, I. (2016, October 17). How the housing boom is remaking Australia's social class structure. *The Conversation*. https://theconversation.com/how-the-housing-boom-is-remaking-australias-social-class-structure-66976.

Yates, Y., & Bradbury, B. (2010). Home ownership as a (crumbling) fourth pillar of social insurance in Australia. *Journal of Housing and the Built Environment, 25*(2), 193–211.

Appendix

Methodology

Most current Australian research into private renting draws on limited demographic and socio-economic data on the characteristics of renter households and there is little information on the social and psychological dimensions of private renting. We commissioned a face-to-face questionnaire survey of 600 private renters in Sydney and Melbourne, Australia's two largest cities accounting for about 40% of the country's population.[1] The survey was designed to capture 200 long-term private renters (ten years or more) and 400 tenants who had been renting for less than ten years. The surveys were undertaken in the private renters' homes in early 2015. Besides interrogating the demographics and employment status of household members, the survey asked respondents about the quality and condition of their accommodation, the terms and condition of their tenancy, their relationship with the landlord or agent who manages their property and perceptions of security of tenure, the rent and affordability of their dwelling and future housing plans.

In order to achieve a sample broadly representative of all private renters in the two cities, respondents were sampled in six areas that were selected using the Australian Bureau of Statistics SA2 geography to represent inner, middle and outer suburban locations. These locations also demonstrably represented high-rent, medium-rent and low-rent housing markets (defined in relation to respective city-wide rent distributions). This approach was considered particularly important in facilitating an investigation of the extent to which the private rental experience varied in different geographic and housing market contexts.

Data sources used to select the fieldwork areas and sample addresses within these areas included the ABS Census of Population and Housing 2011, and state government Rental Bond Board records. Incorporating all private rental tenancies in existence at any given time, these latter address-level data-sets were ideal for our purpose. A random sample of 2,996 private rental property addresses was issued to a market

[1]Funding for the survey and the interviews with long-term private renters was obtained from the Australian Research Council.

A. Morris et al., *The Private Rental Sector in Australia*,
https://doi.org/10.1007/978-981-33-6672-5

research company to generate 600 face-to-face interviews. Quotas were issued to ensure that at least 200 interviewees were long-term renters (ten years or more). In practice, this proved unproblematic and 218 long-term renters were surveyed of 600 in total.

Relating the number of issued addresses to the number of interviews achieved implies a (minimum) response rate of 20%. The actual response rate may have been higher, but since the proportion of addresses at which calls were made was unfortunately not recorded we cannot be specific on this. A low response rate increases the risk that the achieved sample is less than fully representative of the population. As a check on this, referencing 2011census data for the relevant SA2s, we compared the profile of the achieved sample with the recorded profile of the private rental populations of the relevant areas. In most respects there was relatively little difference. For example, the proportion of overseas born respondents in our achieved sample was 62% compared with 64% as recorded in the census. Similarly, the proportion of family households in our sample was 34% compared with 28% in census. And discounting unclassifiable cases, the survey found 33% lacked any tertiary qualification, as compared with 34% in the census. On the same basis, however, the proportion of survey respondents reporting a university qualification was 55% compared with 41% in the census. This may indicate that the respondents were slightly weighted towards higher status households by comparison with the profile of a wholly representative sample. This could have had some influence on the survey findings and should be taken into account when interpreting these. A check against 2011 Census data for Sydney and Melbourne suggests that our sample may have slightly over-represented family households and slightly under-represented renters occupying separate houses by comparison with the combined city-wide private renter/private rental property profiles. However, since the differences were relatively small it was decided to work with unweighted data.

The questionnaire survey was used to recruit interviewees for in-depth interviews. We focused on long-term renters. Survey respondents were asked if they were prepared to be interviewed face-to-face. Sixty semi-structured in-depth interviews were undertaken by the research team in 2015–2016, with the sample evenly split between the two cities and between high, medium and low rent localities within each city. The semi-structured interviews were conducted in the homes of long-term renters. The interviews investigated why interviewees had become long-term renters, their perceptions of security and control, landlord-tenant relations, their sense of home, the broader impacts of being a long-term renter and their future housing plans. All the interviews were audio-recorded and transcribed and organised into main themes and sub-themes using NVivo software.

In addition to the interviewees recruited via the survey, 32 older private renters were interviewed in Sydney and regional New South Wales between 2005 and 2015. All of these interviewees were aged 65 or over, living by themselves and dependent on the government Age Pension solely or primarily for their income. The recruitment of the older private renters was a major challenge. This was mainly due to them being dispersed, isolated and less engaged with organisations. Word of mouth was crucial, as was an advertisement for the study placed in a widely circulated free seniors publication.

The interviews with the older private renters were initially conducted for a project that examined the impact of housing tenure on older Australians reliant on the Age Pension for their income (see Morris, 2016). The interviews focused on their housing histories, the condition and suitability of their accommodation, the cost of the accommodation and its impact on their everyday life and health. The cost of their accommodation was a pivotal focus as it became evident that many of the older private renters were in dire straits due to their rent accounting for much of their Age Pension.

All of the interviews were audio-recorded with consent (ethics permission was obtained from the respective universities of the authors) and fully transcribed. NVivo software was used to facilitate analysis of the interview data.

Reference

Morris, A. (2016). *The Australian Dream: Housing experiences of older Australians.* Melbourne: CSIRO Publishing.

Name Index

A. Morris et al., *The Private Rental Sector in Australia*,
https://doi.org/10.1007/978-981-33-6672-5

Subject Index

A. Morris et al., *The Private Rental Sector in Australia*,
https://doi.org/10.1007/978-981-33-6672-5

The manufacturer's authorised representative in the EU is Springer Nature Customer Service Centre GmbH, Europaplatz 3, 69115 Heidelberg, Germany. If you have any concerns regarding our products, please contact ProductSafety@springernature.com

Printed and bound by CPI Group (UK) Ltd, Croydon, CR0 4YY
30/09/2026
02225264-0020